This is a remarkable book. Karen Fine has a deep and intuitive understanding of narrative medicine and has applied this to veterinary practice in a way that is wise, compassionate and realistic. Dr. Fine pays close attention to the complex dynamics that can exist between client, animal and veterinarian and how to harness these for effective treatment. Her book offers a feast of ideas, tips and heartwarming stories to guide everyday practice. This is an essential read for every veterinary student and practitioner.

— **John Launer**, Health Education England, author of *Narrative-Based Practice in Health and Social Care* (Routledge, 2018)

This innovative book makes a compelling case for reimagining modern veterinary practice in ways that benefit the animal patient, its human caretaker, and veterinary professionals. As human-animal connections evolve, so must the practice of veterinary medicine. Pets today are often considered family members, and scientific advances offer more treatment options to consider. On the other hand, the practice of modern veterinary medicine is increasingly impersonal for both clients and veterinary staff. One remedy, the author suggests, is applying the narrative medicine or "three-dimensional medicine" model, which takes into account the animal patient, the human caregiver, and environment and other contextual aspects. The author, a seasoned veterinarian, skillfully weaves together concepts and methods of the growing narrative medicine movement in human medicine to veterinary practice, as well as insights from history, psychology, and other disciplines. Most compelling, though, are veterinary professionals' stories about their own experiences. Well organized and clearly written, this very readable book is an important resource for veterinary education and practice. It will also appeal to a broad audience of animal lovers and pet owners interested in better understanding of human-animal relationships and veterinary medicine.

— **Carolyn E. Ware**, Associate Professor of English, Louisiana State University, USA

Dr. Fine beautifully describes veterinary narrative medicine in this wide-ranging must-have book for all clinicians. She provides anecdotes that illustrate how applying this approach can improve the care we provide to our patients and clients, while also taking better care of ourselves. She makes the excellent case that narrative medicine is a necessary parallel to evidence-based medicine and makes us better (and more efficient) veterinarians with deeper connections to our clients, patients and work, mitigating pervasive burnout, perfectionism and self-judgement.

— **Annie Wayne**, DVM, MPH, DACVECC, Assistant Professor, Emergency and Critical Care, Cummings School of Veterinary Medicine, Tufts University

Dr. Karen Fine was the one to introduce me this last year to the concept of narrative medicine. I realize through our conversations and in the lessons learned from reading her book that this is an incredibly powerful way to navigate building community, decreasing empathic distress and compassion fatigue, and practicing veterinary medicine in a sustainable way. This book provides an invaluable learning opportunity for all stages of veterinary professional development. Dr. Fine's voice and choice of words struck just the right balance between wise instructor and caring friend making the reading so enjoyable. Her work supports an important contribution to the necessary shift of our professional culture that sees the people as much as the veterinary patients with compassion and care.

— **Sonja A. Olson**, DVM, Clinical Health and Well-being Trainer at BluePearl Veterinary Partners, USA

By bringing attention to the human component of veterinary medicine, Dr. Fine has provided us with an empathic and holistic perspective to medical care that has great potential for healing in the animal community; not only for animals, but their human companions and veterinary professionals as well.

— **Julie Gass**, MSW, LICSW, Angell Animal Medical Center, USA

Narrative medicine is a concept thoroughly laid out here by Dr. Karen Fine to consider the whole picture, the important human/animal bond, and the well-being of the entire unit. There, in so doing, the veterinarian is also encouraged to be self-compassionate and embrace their humanity in their valued roles as caregivers to the animals of this partnership. This book's wisdom comes from a place of experience, tenderness, and "you are doing it right already" crafting. There is fair acknowledgement of the heavy parts, to the role of the peace-bringers we can be, and to the necessity that we veterinarians take as good care of ourselves as we do our animal patients.

— **Monica Mansfield**, D.V.M., Chairperson of MVMA Wellness Committee and MVMA President-Elect

Narrative Medicine in Veterinary Practice

Improving Client Communication, Patient Care, and Veterinary Well-Being

Karen R. Fine

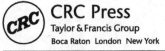

CRC Press
Taylor & Francis Group
Boca Raton London New York

CRC Press is an imprint of the
Taylor & Francis Group, an **informa** business

First edition published 2022
by CRC Press
6000 Broken Sound Parkway NW, Suite 300, Boca Raton, FL 33487-2742

and by CRC Press
2 Park Square, Milton Park, Abingdon, Oxon, OX14 4RN

© 2022 Karen R. Fine

CRC Press is an imprint of Taylor & Francis Group, LLC

Reasonable efforts have been made to publish reliable data and information, but the author and publisher cannot assume responsibility for the validity of all materials or the consequences of their use. The authors and publishers have attempted to trace the copyright holders of all material reproduced in this publication and apologize to copyright holders if permission to publish in this form has not been obtained. If any copyright material has not been acknowledged, please write and let us know so we may rectify in any future reprint.

Except as permitted under U.S. Copyright Law, no part of this book may be reprinted, reproduced, transmitted, or utilized in any form by any electronic, mechanical, or other means, now known or hereafter invented, including photocopying, microfilming, and recording, or in any information storage or retrieval system, without written permission from the publishers.

For permission to photocopy or use material electronically from this work, access www.copyright.com or contact the Copyright Clearance Center, Inc. (CCC), 222 Rosewood Drive, Danvers, MA 01923, 978-750-8400. For works that are not available on CCC, please contact mpkbookspermissions@tandf.co.uk

Trademark notice: Product or corporate names may be trademarks or registered trademarks and are used only for identification and explanation without intent to infringe.

ISBN: 978-0-367-64763-6 (hbk)
ISBN: 978-0-367-64761-2 (pbk)
ISBN: 978-1-003-12613-3 (ebk)

DOI: 10.1201/9781003126133

Typeset in Sabon
by codeMantra

In loving memory of my grandfather "Oupa," Maurice Fine, MD

Contents

Introduction

Veterinary medicine has changed dramatically over the past 50 years. Pets are openly considered "family members" by many, and far more diagnostics and treatments are available for them. While solo practitioners exist, in many regions they are no longer the norm. Clinics often employ multiple doctors and many are corporately owned. Certified technicians, once rare, have taken over growing roles. Computer records are replacing paper records, and many practices interface with clients through email, text, or website apps. While many of these changes are positive (or at least have positive aspects), they can also lead to a less personal experience for the client as well as the practitioner. Compared to the days of British veterinarian and author Alf Wight, who wrote as James Herriott, the medicine may be more advanced, but the relationships with our clients are often more removed.

Human medicine has been faced with many of the same circumstances over the past several decades, and the field of narrative medicine has arisen partly as a response to these issues (Charon 2006, 6–9).

Narrative medicine could also be called three-dimensional medicine. Medicine practiced in two dimensions considers the patient as an example of a disease (i.e., the Westie in Room 2 with chronic skin allergies). Medicine practiced in three dimensions sees not only the patient, but also the caregiver (client), as well as the dog's environment, diet, and history. The patient now has a name, a context, a *story*. This particular Westie, "Conrad," may live with a chronically ill owner, Mary, who is unable to bathe him, although the bathing helps his skin. Conrad may also be impacted by Mary's stress and fatigue. You may be able to work with Mary to come up with helpful strategies to benefit your patient, but only after openly listening to Mary and what she has to say.

Considering a wider view of a patient might feel overwhelming, but narrative medicine gives us the tools to make it manageable, allowing us to pinpoint our questioning to diagnose and treat our patients more easily, and often more successfully. How can we best interact with our clients to get the information we need? How can we explain our concerns and recommendations to them? Is it possible to overcome inherent biases for certain clients, or to act mindfully when we are stressed or rushed? This book addresses these questions and hopes to provide a way to maintain and even expand the intimate experience of the family doctor for both client and practitioner.

But that sounds complicated, you may be thinking. *I don't have time to make every encounter into a story.* Yet a narrative does not need to be complicated. A single-frame cartoon tells a story. A photo tells a story, as does a painting or a song. Stories are how people have understood the world around us for thousands of years. Stories are all around us, including the television and movies we watch and the social media we post and follow. There is a reason we "read" a radiograph.

Stories are also present in our work environment, and our staff members hold a wealth of information about our patients and clients. Involving staff members in the practice of narrative medicine is essential, as they are often the ones to alert us to information crucial to our decision making. Staff members are also part of our own narratives as practitioners, as members of our "work family." And, staff members grieve with us over the loss of a patient they may have known for years.

Narrative medicine is rooted in the history of medicine: what does it mean to *doctor*, as a verb (Charon 2006)? Human medicine has traditionally reflected more upon this than our profession, perhaps due to treating patients of our own species, who can consider and discuss their own mortality. Veterinary medicine is arguably more hands-on than human medicine; we get dirty, we get down on the floor. We get the job done, but there is little room for contemplation. Reflection has not been traditionally emphasized, taught, or encouraged in veterinary medical training, yet it is something all practitioners may benefit from. Many of us reflect upon something only when we do not achieve a desired outcome: the patient died – what could I have done differently? Reflection, sadly, is often tied to shame in our profession. However, it should not and does not have to be this way. Reflection is a helpful practice that can allow us to become better doctors and increase the wellness in our profession.

Grief is a regular feature in the practice of veterinary medicine. As doctors, we are trained to problem-solve, yet we cannot solve the pain of loss. Narrative medicine offers some ideas for ourselves, our clients, and our staff to address the often overlooked toll that grief can take upon our lives.

Practitioner wellness has been a recent focus due to the awareness of suicide in our profession, and narrative medicine can help us here as well. This book explores how our own narratives and those of our patients/clients can be viewed as a Venn diagram of overlapping circles, which we can slide apart if we become overly invested in a relationship or outcome and it begins to affect our mental health. The text also introduces something called the Connection Triangle, unique to veterinary medicine, which considers our relationship with the human-animal bond as well as our patients and clients.

The book draws from two leaders in the field of human narrative medicine: Dr. Rita Charon from Columbia School of Medicine, author of *Narrative Medicine*, and Dr. John Launer of the Tavistok clinic in the United Kingdom, author of *Narrative-Based Primary Care, a Practical Guide*. In order to pursue her interest in the ways a narrative focus could help the practice of medicine, Dr. Charon turned to the field of literature, obtaining a PhD in English. She first wrote about narrative medicine in a landmark paper in *JAMA* in 2001, effectively initiating the field in the United States (Charon 2001). Dr. Charon invented something she terms the Parallel Chart, written in parallel with a clinical record, to help increase reflection and understanding of narrative medicine (Charon 2006). Dr. Launer, also seeking to further his understanding and work, turned to the field of psychology and family therapy, codeveloping a model of interactional skills called "Conversations Inviting Change" (Launer 2002, 22–32). While the approaches of the two clinicians are different, their goals align, and veterinary medicine has much to learn from both styles of teaching and practice.

I'm also going to draw from my own experience, which includes over 20 years of house call practice, and nearly as many years of practicing conventional veterinary medicine integrated with traditional Chinese veterinary medicine (TCVM), including acupuncture.

I have chosen a format for Part II of the book that follows along a typical small animal appointment. I will explore how, from a narrative medicine perspective, a practitioner can prepare themselves for an appointment, conduct the interview through the interaction with the client and patient and exam procedure, and write up the report afterward.

Veterinary narrative medicine is a new field, and we thus have an opportunity to define it moving forward. How might this approach help our profession with its problems, and its practitioners with their needs? How could it improve both our professional and personal lives? By considering these questions, we may contribute to the development of veterinary narrative medicine over time. It is my hope that, in addition to learning ways to increase their enjoyment and enrichment of veterinary medical practice, readers will recognize themselves and others in these pages and realize they may already have been practicing narrative medicine.

Author

Dr. Karen Fine's interest in narrative medicine stems from many years of doing home visits, her experience as a holistic, integrative practitioner, and her love of reading. She achieved certification in veterinary acupuncture in 2002 and is a graduate of the Mindfulness Based Stress Reduction (MBSR) program. Dr. Fine is an adjunct professor at the Cummings School of Veterinary Medicine at Tufts University. Her forthcoming memoir, *The Other Family Doctor*, is being published by Anchor books, a division of Penguin Random House.

Narrative Medicine in Human Medical Practice

CHAPTER ONE

Overview of Narrative Medicine

Narrative medicine (NM) isn't new – it's been practiced for as long as there have been health practitioners caring for patients. The ability to see the patient as a unique individual with a specific story has long played a part in medical practice. As medical care has grown more impersonal, however, there have been decreased opportunities for human connections and fewer chances for practitioners to connect with their patient's story.

In this chapter, we explore the field of NM in human medical practice, including how it is practiced and taught. We also focus on the work of two leaders in the field, Dr. Rita Charon in the United States and Dr. John Launer in the United Kingdom.

Key Points

- Narrative medicine (NM) is a fast-growing approach in human medicine that is practiced formally in many countries and includes many different but complementary ideas and philosophies.
- NM can improve communication skills, patient outcomes, and practitioner well-being.
- Medical schools try to graduate physicians with "narrative competence."
- Much of the field of human NM can be adapted for use in veterinary medicine.

DOI: 10.1201/9781003126133-2

What is Narrative Medicine?

In her book, *Narrative Medicine: Honoring the Stories of Illness*, Dr. Rita Charon describes a critically ill elderly patient she cared for as an intern.

> He was irretrievably sick, bed-bound for months, with…a serious infection in the blood, and his kidneys were failing. Multiple strokes had left him comatose for many months in the nursing home. And yet his wife sat at his bed all day, every day. I remember her tasteful blouse and her pearls. She would ask me every day, 'Is he going to be all right?'

Dr. Charon describes her feelings of isolation and helplessness.

> We were in it, together, we three—this gravely ill man trying so hard to die, his wife bereft by his loss and unable to fathom her life without him, and me, the intern, who wanted like crazy to save him…What I did not know how to do for my patient and his wife was to get to the heart of their suffering. I knew how to manage the man's fluid status and antibiotics, and I even knew, more or less, when to call a halt to aggressive care, but I did not know how to manage the fact of his dying. I did not know how to manage his wife's fear and loss. Nor did I know what to do with my own suffering in the face of theirs.
> (Charon 2006, 33–34)

NM considers the aspects of medicine beyond fluid status and the prescribing of medications; beyond the differential diagnosis and prognosis to understand the patient and connect with them. Once the patient's narrative is understood, it becomes easier to work together toward a treatment plan addressing their unique needs. NM also allows us to consider our own stories and how they affect and are impacted by our work.

Current Overview

NM is studied in medical and nursing schools around the world. In the United States, Columbia University is the center. The extensive program, created and led by Dr. Charon, offers both a certificate and a master's degree in NM, as well as workshops throughout the year. The field is sometimes called narrative-based medicine, or medical humanities (especially in Europe).

Colleges and universities with programs in NM, typically affiliated with medical schools, include the University of Toronto, King's College London, the University of Kentucky, the University of Southern California, Boston University, the University of Arizona College of Medicine – Phoenix, Lewis Katz School of

Medicine at Temple University, and Wake Forest University. In addition, many medical schools offer programs connected with a medical humanities curriculum, including Stanford and Yale.

There are several NM journals, including *Literature and Medicine* (Johns Hopkins), *Intima, Bellevue Literary Review, Chronicles of Narrative Medicine* based in Italy, and a more informal online magazine called *Pulse*, where doctors, patients, and other medical professionals tell their stories. There are NM societies all over the world, including the newly formed European Narrative Medicine Society, EUNAMES.

Numerous books and journal articles have been written about NM. For this book, I have chosen to focus on the works of two of the field's leaders: Dr. Rita Charon in the United States and Dr. John Launer in the United Kingdom. Both have published extensively on the topic and are internationally recognized experts in NM.

The following story illustrates how NM can assist veterinarians and how comparable our professional demands are to those of physicians; note the similarities to Dr. Charon's story at the beginning of this chapter.

Case Story: *In Search of the Story,* by Dr. Annie Wayne

One of the drivers for me to change and increase communications training for our veterinary students at Tufts came from an experience as a new intern. I was in my first week of my internship at Angell, working overnights, and one of my first cases was an older woman with an older cat presenting for not eating. Point-of-care bloodwork showed that the cat was in renal failure. As I looked over the bloodwork and prepared to enter the room, I felt completely unprepared. I knew the medicine and what the options were, but I felt completely unprepared for how to help the owner navigate making a decision for her cat. As I reflect back on the situation now, I realize how powerful NM is to have as a framework for these discussions. What I really needed in that moment was the understanding that I needed to hear from the owner what her story was, so I could help her decide whether to spend several thousand dollars to hospitalize her geriatric cat with an uncertain outcome or help her say goodbye.

Focus: Dr. Rita Charon

NM effectively began in the United States after the *Journal of the American Medical Association* (JAMA) published a landmark paper by Dr. Rita Charon in 2001. Entitled *Narrative Medicine: A Model for Empathy, Reflection, Profession, and Trust*, the paper discusses Dr. Charon's relationship with a patient and examines some key concerns. She describes "four of medicine's central narrative situations: those between physician and patient, physician and self, physician and colleagues, and physicians and society" (Charon 2001). In veterinary medicine, we would add those between physician and client. These terms are important because NM is not solely about listening to the stories of our patients/clients; it is also about our own stories and how they fit into our practices and our lives, as well as our relationships with our colleagues and the larger society.

Another oft-quoted line from the paper reads,

> Along with scientific ability, physicians need the ability to listen to the narratives of the patient, grasp and honor their meanings, and be moved to act on the patient's behalf. This is narrative competence, that is, the competence that human beings use to absorb, interpret and respond to stories
>
> (Charon 2001)

Narrative competence has become a commonly used term in NM programs in medical schools and other school curricula, with the goal being to graduate practitioners with narrative competence.

In her book, *Narrative Medicine: Honoring the Stories of Illness*, Dr. Charon describes the study of medicine as being based on generalities (i.e., *most patients...*), while the practice of medicine involving an individual patient necessitates analyzing a unique individual's particular details (*this patient...*) (Charon 2006, p. 9). The same applies to veterinary medicine; as clinicians, we must determine what is going on in the patient in front of us, not the animals written about in a journal article or book chapter. Diseases present differently in distinct individuals, test results vary, and the effects of medications are different in different bodies. NM emphasizes treating patients as individuals, rather than as representatives of their diseases and conditions.

Dr. Charon emphasizes the importance of reflection in medical practice, and she invented a tool for this purpose called a "parallel chart," in which an experience can be written about reflectively in parallel with the medical chart (Charon 2006, 155).

Reflective writing workshops are a hallmark of the NM program utilized by Dr. Charon, the NM program at Columbia University Narrative Medicine, and many other NM programs. These are short (typically 1 hour) workshops to practice close listening. The workshops involve a discussion followed by a short session of reflective writing to a prompt, the results of which are then shared in small groups (Winkel 2016). One list of workshops for obstetrics/gynecology residents involves such themes as work-life balance, death and dying, managing expectations, coping mechanisms, professionalism and humility, friendship and boundaries, and making mistakes (Winkel 2016).

Dr. Charon has separated the physician encounter into three parts, which she terms attention, representation, and affiliation.

Attention, Representation, Affiliation

Attention

Dr. Charon's triad of the NM encounter begins with attention; as she states, "we must begin our care by listening to the patient's account of what has occurred and confirming our reception of the report (Charon 2006, 132)." Attention does not simply mean paying just enough attention to confirm your suspicion of what is going on, or only listening to part of what the person is saying. Attention means giving the patient – or in the case of veterinary medicine, the patient *and* the client – your *full and complete* attention. To do this, Charon describes the skill of close listening, or listening attentively. Close listening, Charon maintains, is a skill that can be taught by practicing the related skill of close reading, learning to read a story while paying full attention to the narrative as well as the narrative process: what is left unsaid, how it is framed, how the narrator affects the story. Mindfulness is another way to help a clinician learn to pay attention, by being able to tune out distractions and focus fully on the person's story (Charon 2006, 132).

Representation

Once close attention has been paid to the story, the next step is representation. The story is both interpreted and told through the lens of the practitioner. After hearing the same story, different clinicians will represent that story in different ways; representation is not about replicating a narrative, but about interpreting a narrative in good faith, after paying close attention. Practitioners are unable to separate themselves from the narratives they represent. Representation may involve writing in the medical chart, reflective writing such as in a parallel chart, and acting upon the information collected from the client/patient.

Affiliation

Dr. Charon describes affiliation as the "outcome" of narrative work – a community-building connection.

> We live through victories and defeats with our patients; we are moved by these events as they happen; we incur ethical duties toward them; and we become different people ourselves because of them.
>
> (Charon 2006, 151)

Attention and representation allow us to connect with our clients in a deeper way as we work together toward a common goal, the optimum health of our patients.

Focus: Dr. John Launer

While Dr. Charon turned to literature and the arts to study NM, Dr. Launer turned to the field of social work, specifically family therapy. Dr. Launer has focused his training seminars and courses on post-graduate medical education, where he emphasizes "microskills" based on the "Conversations Inviting Change" framework outlined below. He has found that "people who acquired narrative skills through doing peer supervision on our courses became more proficient in applying these to their work with patients and clients." (Launer 2018, xiii).

Dr. Launer offers a wonderful description of NM: the idea that a patient arrives for an appointment accompanied by a certain narrative, and that, together with the physician, a new narrative is cocreated. "Instead of being a fixer or an adviser, the clinician becomes a questioner and a proposer of reframed stories," Launer writes (Launer 2002, 23).

The skills outlined below can help address the following dilemmas Dr. Launer has identified, which affect many professions:

- How do you practice when the authority of professionals, including doctors and social workers, can no longer be taken for granted?
- How can you share power with patients and clients, without letting go of evidence and best practice?
- How do you work alongside colleagues with other professions, views, beliefs, and priorities?
- How can you be a care professional and remain a caring person? (Launer 2018, xiii–xiv)

The following section is an excerpt from Dr. Launer's 2018 book, *Narrative-Based Practice in Health and Social Care.*

Conversations Inviting Change – The Seven C's

Conversations. Effective conversations don't just describe reality, they create new understanding of it. Conversations can be seen as interventions in their own right: the end as well as the means. Simply by taking place, they create opportunities for people to rethink and redefine their realities.

Curiosity. This is what turns conversations from chatter into something more substantial. It invites others to reframe their stories in different ways. An essential aspect of curiosity is aspiring to neutrality (to individuals, to blame, to interpretations, to facts). Curiosity should also extend to yourself. What are your own thoughts about the interaction? How can you become curious about your own biases and prejudices, or prevent yourself being critical or impatient? How does your role or power limit the kind of neutrality you can offer?

Contexts. This is what it is most effective to be curious about. Important contexts in work with patients and clients are families, cultures, beliefs, and faith. In conversations between practitioners, they include teams, organizations and professional networks, hierarchies, history, geography, and belief systems and values.

Complexity. Rather than looking for a "quick fix" in every situation, it is better to consider any problem as part of an infinite and unpredictable dance of interactions. A sense of complexity gets away from fixed ideas of cause and effect, unchangeable problems, and over-concrete solutions. Instead, it emphasizes ideas such as emergence, evolution, and gradual resolution.

Challenge. Professional conversations can be seen as a form of shared activity, in which one person is challenging another to think of a different description of what is going on. What you are looking for is a better account of reality than the present one, which means a way of narrating the story that makes better sense for others of what they are going through, and may include practical actions.

Caution. You need to use sensitivity, and monitor your own emotional responses, to make sure you are matching your words to suit the other person and their capacity to extend their thinking at that moment. If someone wants straightforward information and advice, be prepared to give it (while being aware of the limitations of doing so without an opportunity for the other person to make sense of it for themselves). Also, remember you're not doing therapy – on colleagues or on patients!

Care. The role of health and social care professionals is to look after others. None of the ideas and techniques will work unless you are respectful, affectionate, and attentive. Narrative-based practice needs to be grounded in moral commitment (Launer 2018, 37–38).

Relationship to Evidence-Based Medicine

Evidence-based medicine (EBM) was originally defined as "the conscientious, explicit, and judicious use of current best evidence in making decisions about the care of individual patients" (Sackett 1996). What is EBM's relationship to NM?

The EBM movement first began in human medicine and has faced further scrutiny and review there than in veterinary medicine. While the goal of utilizing the best possible evidence when making treatment decisions is admirable, EBM has in effect created a hierarchical system which values certain evidence above others, and some physicians believe it has become a dogmatic and overused approach (Meier and Nietlispach 2019; Charon and Wyer 2008). One article states, "In the minds of many, a laudatory mantra chanting of EBM immediately gives legitimacy to whatever falls under its umbrella" (Jenicek 2006). Others lament the lack of evidence that EBM has led to improved patient care and question the role of the pharmaceutical industry in deciding which trials to run, which can potentially result in lopsided evidence (Every-Palmer and Howick 2014). In addition, a lack of evidence does not mean a treatment is ineffective. "Good evidence is often lacking in medicine…Lack of evidence of effectiveness does not prove ineffectiveness" (Woolf and George 2000).

Not every treatment lends itself easily to the EBM model. In veterinary medicine, the field of veterinary acupuncture provides an example. Acupuncture is considered "proven effective" by the World Health Organization for numerous human conditions and is utilized by hundreds, if not thousands, of veterinarians worldwide who have undergone intensive training. Yet a shortage of EBM has been misused as an argument to claim that veterinary acupuncture is ineffective (Magalhães-Sant'Ana 2019). Veterinary acupuncturists have voiced a desire for more evidence-based research on acupuncture in animals (Shmalberg and Memon 2015). The lack of studies such as randomized controlled trials (RCT) is based upon two fundamental issues. First, who would pay for the studies? There are no profitable pharmaceutical companies involved. Second, optimal results from acupuncture occur when each treatment is individualized, and research data would need to be interpreted accordingly. A refusal to consider therapies which do not fit neatly into models such as the RCT misinterprets the spirit of EBM and could deny patients access to treatments and care many veterinarians find effective.

EBM seems to exist in opposition to the humble anecdote, a singular story which may or may not represent a repeatable or universal experience. Yet practice occurs through stories, the telling and explaining of symptoms and contexts, the discovery of disease, the navigation through its course, and the connection of patient (or client) and practitioner. Clinicians discuss cases, sharing their success stories with one another and seeking advice on difficult scenarios; such case discussions are termed "curbside consultations" in human medicine and are arguably an important part of medical practice (Cook et al. 2014). Most practitioners understand that what works for one individual may not help another, and medicine cannot be best practiced through a one-size-fits-all approach. Clinically relevant data will always be an important part of the practice of medicine, but it cannot be the entirety of medicine.

There is a growing movement in human medicine to find a balance between the approaches of EBM and NM (Kosko et al. 2006). Columbia University has introduced a program titled "narrative evidence-based medicine", which Dr. Charon writes "recognizes the narrative features of *all* data and the evidentiary status of *all* clinical text (Charon and Wyer 2008)." The integration of the two approaches recognizes that they do not exist in opposition to one another, but in harmony. The Yin–Yang symbol provides an excellent illustration of this relationship.

The Yin–Yang symbol represents a type of dichotomy that may be unfamiliar to some people. The black and white parts do not represent matters that are good/bad, right/wrong, or either/or. Instead, they represent mutually dependent entities: one cannot exist without the other. Day follows night, just as warm is relative to cold. The focus is on *balance*, as problems happen when the two sides are out of balance with one another. A deficiency on one side will lead to an excess on another, and vice versa.

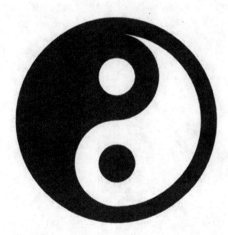

EBM – or, more broadly, the best clinically relevant data – and NM exist in such a state. They are mutually beneficial, and both are often necessary to provide the best possible medical care.

What does this look like in practice? It means utilizing evidence-based medicine without a dogmatic adherence to it, maintaining an awareness of its shortcomings, and not allowing the best available evidence to consistently override clinical experience and judgment. It means allowing ample space for the practitioner's creativity and ability to address the needs of patients and clients with individualized solutions. Ultimately, it means recognizing the practice of medicine as an art as well as a science, and understanding that while much is known about medical evidence, there is also much we have to learn.

Suggestions for Reflection and Discussion

- Have you ever had an experience like Dr. Wayne's and Dr. Charon's?
- Choose one of the "seven C's" and think about it during a client interaction. Did it change your idea of what was going on during the conversation?
- Can you add anything to the list of seven C's?
- How do you relate evidence-based medicine to NM?

CHAPTER TWO

Related Fields

What are the roots of narrative medicine (NM) in medical practice? NM is related to several other fields, and an exploration of these disciplines will contribute to a broader understanding of NM, the scope of its use in human medicine, and its potential for veterinary medicine.

Key Points

- While NM may be most closely related to the field of communications, it has close ties to many other disciplines.
- NM provides a way to explore ethics and philosophy, which have not traditionally been well explored in veterinary medicine.
- The humanities can help clinicians increase their curiosity and observational skills, foster compassion, and support the tolerance of ambiguity and uncertainty.
- Mindfulness skills can help develop practitioner focus, which can lead to improved patient care and client communication.
- An understanding of basic sociology and psychology can improve veterinarian's understanding of our clients as well as our patients.

Communications

Narrative medicine (NM) is perhaps most easily compared to the field of communications. In both human and veterinary medicine, communication has evolved from the days when doctors gave their diagnoses and prescriptions in a top-down manner with minimal feedback from patients or clients. However, many

DOI: 10.1201/9781003126133-3

believe the practice of medicine has been dehumanized, and NM has grown out of a desire to improve medical care while also increasing practitioner well-being (Charon, Narrative Medicine, Honoring the Stories of Illness 2006, 6–7). NM expands upon the basic communication skills taught in both medical and veterinary schools in line with the Calgary Cambridge model to provide an intuitive framework for goals and methods of enhanced communication.

In a large study of veterinarians in the United States and the United Kingdom, 98% of respondents agreed that communication skills were as important as or more important than clinical knowledge (McDermott et al. 2015). And while an Australian survey of both veterinarians and veterinary students ranked "verbal communication and interpersonal skills as the most important skill set for an entry-level veterinarian (Haldane et al. 2017)," training in communication has been found to be "very limited" and "lacking" according to a large review study which "identified a gap in the communication skills of veterinary professionals (Pun 2020)."

As this book illustrates, NM is far more than an expanded communications curriculum or program. Rather, it is an exploration of the creative "arts" aspect of our work which is essential to integrate with the "scientific" practice of medicine. NM can help practitioners communicate with clients, colleagues, staff members, and themselves.

Ethics and Philosophy

Human medicine has enjoyed a long history of reflection, helped in part by the field of medical humanities, explored in the following section. NM has informed the field of medical ethics by providing an approach for reflection on many aspects of medical care. By paying attention to the patient's story, NM allows the practitioner to reflect upon how that story may continue and how can the practitioner best contribute to the unique story of their patient? NM also allows for the practitioner's own reflection; how did this patient's story affect my own story? NM is an approach that allows veterinary medicine to ask questions historically integral to human medicine such as *What is life? What is suffering? How have I changed after encountering this patient?* Such questions do not easily lend themselves to controlled double-blinded studies or anatomy textbooks. Rather, they may be best understood through the explorations of narratives.

In his book *Being Mortal: Medicine and What Matters in the End*, Dr. Atul Gawande discusses how modern medicine has changed patient care. Instead of a person living until they became seriously ill and dying quickly, many people are now able to live with chronic illnesses despite potential changes in their quality of life (Gawande 2014, 25–29). The same is true in veterinary medicine, and the field has changed dramatically over the past several decades regarding options for patient care. As a result, after working together to resolve or manage multiple medical issues over the course of an animal's life, many pet owners develop a close bond with their veterinarian. Pet owners may also experience closer bonds with their animals after caring for them through multiple medical events. The veterinary profession has only begun to consider the impact of these changes.

Moral stress, or the response of the practitioner to facing ethical dilemmas in the course of practice, has been suggested as a primary trigger for compassion fatigue (Kahler 2015) and may be expanded due to these closer relationships between client and animal and client and veterinarian. NM has the potential to help veterinary medicine reflect upon and explore these ethical situations, which are only beginning to be widely discussed. At the heart of many ethical veterinary dilemmas lies the dual duties we have to our patients and our clients. As practice owner Dr. Eileen Mulcahy states, "I am often in conflict between my responsibility to my patient versus my obligation to my client." Small wonder, then, that the responsibility of veterinarians to their own well-being often comes last. NM offers a way to explore these ethical issues and support practitioners as we consider our changing profession.

Medical Humanities

Human medicine has the advantage of the medical humanities, a field encompassing the broad intersection of art and medicine, including literature, art, music, and theater. Along with the fields of ethics and philosophy discussed earlier, the field of medical humanities examines questions such as *What is the role of a doctor in a patient's life? How does society view illness? How has that changed over time?* Also considered are issues related to what is termed "the human condition:" birth, illness, suffering, death. The study of medical humanities fosters skills vital to medical practice such as compassion, reflection, the ability to pay mindful attention to the stories of patients, and the ability to "read between the lines" of those stories (Mangione et al. 2018). The study of medical humanities also offers a way to explore the ethics and philosophy of medicine while being removed from the realities of patient care. Physician and author Dr. Danielle Ofri writes,

> While medical students often fear the avalanche of knowledge they are required to learn during training, it is learning to translate that knowledge into wisdom that is the greatest challenge of becoming a doctor. Part of that challenge is learning to tolerate ambiguity and uncertainty, a difficult feat for doctors who are taught to question anything that is not evidence based or peer reviewed. The medical humanities specialize in this ambiguity

and uncertainty, which are hallmarks of actual clinical practice but rarely addressed in medical education. The humanities also force reflection and contemplation-skills that are crucial to thoughtful decision making and to personal wellness...Well integrated, the humanities can be the key to transforming medical knowledge into clinical wisdom.

(Ofri 2017)

Dr. Rita Charon's study of NM began in the field of literature, and the field of human NM at Columbia emphasizes the relationship of medical practice to literature and other creative arts. Medical humanities are included in medical school curricula in many countries, including the United States, Canada, the United Kingdom, and Australia (Gordon 2005). One multi-institutional study demonstrated that medical student exposure to the humanities correlated significantly with several positive personal qualities and was strongly inversely correlated with aspects of burnout (Mangione et al. 2018). Another study considered a medical school elective entitled "The Art of Observation" and found that students who had participated in a program involving art museum visits demonstrated enhanced observational skills, improved socialization, and decreased symptoms of burnout (He et al. 2019).

Veterinary medicine has historically not been overly concerned with the human condition, likely because we are one step removed. And while veterinarians are usually compassionate people, self-reflection is not typically modeled or taught in veterinary school. As a result, the profession is, perhaps, overly practical, with a motto that could be described as "get dirty, get it done, and move on." There is little time given to considering *what just happened*, especially in terms of connections with people or animals. However, this is beginning to change, and the focus on veterinary well-being is pushing us to expand our sights. There has even been recent interest in the potential of veterinary humanities; in October 2020, the first online conference for the network of veterinary humanities was held at the University of Vienna in Austria (Network Veterinary Humanities 2020).

Pediatric NM

Pediatrics is the human medical specialty arguably most closely related to veterinary medicine. Like our patients, young children are unable to communicate verbally, may not understand what we or their caretakers want from them, and may exhibit behaviors that make examinations and treatment challenging. In addition, young children must rely on their caretaker both to communicate with medical professionals and for their care at home, including administering medications and managing the environment for optimal health and safety.

Naturally, any comparisons between pediatrics and veterinary medicine must be made with the understanding that pets are not children. Yet, there may be things we can learn from pediatric NM.

An article in the journal *Pediatrics*, entitled *Half as Sad: A Plea for Narrative Medicine in Pediatric Residency Training*, points out how pediatricians lack training on communicating with parents of seriously or terminally ill children. The article states,

> ...a resident may spend an hour sitting with the family of a child newly diagnosed with leukemia, exploring their feelings of guilt and despair, the fear that they had failed to recognize that their child was ill, and their terror about what chemotherapy might bring. At handover, this experience is necessarily reduced to '3-year-old boy, new diagnosis of leukemia. Currently stable. Started induction chemotherapy today. At risk for tumor lysis.' Although we are trained over many years to give concise presentations, we are not trained to process the narrative content of the multifaceted relationships we have with patients and families. This reduction of complex emotional experiences to brief, dispassionate retellings occurs daily. The consequence for the physician may be desensitization or maladaptive behaviors.

The authors have developed a curriculum for training pediatric residents in NM. The title of the article refers to a statement made by a senior physician to a pediatric resident. The resident was simply told that it was his responsibility to "never feel more than 50% as sad as a patient's family" (Diorio and Nowaczyk 2019).

We can also look to pediatrics for research on self-disclosure, discussed in Chapter Five, and discussions with vaccine-hesitant clients, discussed in Chapter Fourteen.

Mindfulness

Dr. Jon Kabat-Zinn, creator of the 8-week mindfulness-based stress reduction (MBSR) program, defines mindfulness as "awareness that arises through paying attention, on purpose, in the present moment, non-judgementally" (Jon Kabat-Zinn: Defining Mindfulness 2017). In medical practice, mindfulness serves to increase our focus on the story in front of us, the one the person is telling us *now*. NM incorporates mindfulness to help us be fully present despite distractions to receive our client's story. Mindful strategies can also be applied to reflective practices to improve practitioner well-being, and we will explore that further in Chapter Thirteen.

Mindfulness has been studied in human health care settings for many years for patients, students, and practitioners, and has applications for improving practitioner performance in addition to enhancing well-being and resilience. After British medical students attended a mindfulness training course, "Students reported a new relationship to their thoughts and feelings which gave a greater sense of control and resiliency, an ability to manage their workload better, and more acceptance of their limitations as learners (Malpass et al. 2019)." A multi-center study which looked at clinicians who had completed the Mindful Attention Awareness Scale found that patients of high-mindfulness clinicians gave higher ratings on clinician communication and overall satisfaction with the visit (Beach et al. 2013). The effects of mindfulness meditation on the brain have been an area of interest, and numerous studies have examined the ways mindfulness practice affects brain structure (Linder 2019).

Mindfulness practice is beginning to be assessed as an intervention to address stress among medical and veterinary students (Pontin et al. 2020). Dr. Kabat-Zinn's MBSR course has been taught around the world to thousands of participants and is the subject of numerous studies. The course teaches participants to focus their attention on the present moment, not the past (should I have treated that patient differently?) or the future (I hope I get out on time tonight).

Psychology, Sociology, and Social work

Psychology and sociology help us better understand not only our animal patients but also our human clients. The study of family systems theory provides an understanding of human behavior, especially when we are dealing with multiple owners with varying perspectives and priorities.

Pet owners may have one or more of a variety of mental illnesses. A needy, high-maintenance client could be suffering from an anxiety disorder, while a client who seems difficult to communicate with might have autism spectrum disorder. A basic understanding of these conditions could improve our interactions and help us not take client behavior personally.

Issues surrounding grief and death are central to our work, and a deeper understanding of the mechanics of grief could benefit most practitioners. While we are not social workers, we need to feel comfortable discussing grief, death, and euthanasia with our clients and coworkers. Ideally, this comfort level should include sustaining a healthy ability to reflect about these issues.

The field of compassion and self-compassion research is a new area which could help us to uncover the differences between compassion and empathy, the potential harms and benefits, and the influence of self-compassion on well-being and resilience.

Veterinary behavior is the closest veterinary field to human psychology, as it incorporates the study of human behavior as well as the behavior of other species to identify how an animal relates to its human environment. For instance, a knowledge of feline elimination behavior in the wild is helpful when discussing the common issue of a cat who refuses to use a litter box. Veterinary behavior is a natural fit for NM, and a consult with a veterinary behaviorist is likely to be thorough and consider the day-to-day life of the patient. Any recommendations given without a clear picture of the animal's home and family situation would likely be less effective.

Finally, the growing field of veterinary social work can guide us as we learn more about the intersection of veterinary medicine and social work.

Holistic and Integrative Medicine

Holistic veterinary medicine encompasses many different types of therapies, including acupuncture, herbal medicine, and homeopathy; it is often combined with Western medicine to be called integrative medicine. Like NM, the hallmark of holistic or integrative care is individualized medicine; the treatment is for an individual, not a disease entity. While holistic medicine is not related to NM per se, their approaches are similar.

Traditional Chinese veterinary medicine (TCVM), which encompasses veterinary acupuncture, involves an entire system of diagnoses as well as treatment. TCVM analyzes the physical body differently than Western medicine, placing greater emphasis on the patient's history to gain a wide-angle view of the animal and its environment. An intake exam for an acupuncture consultation, whether for human or animal, often involves more questions than a Western medical consult. It is, therefore, typical for a first-time acupuncture consult to require more time than subsequent treatments and to be booked and billed accordingly.

This expanded history taking considers multiple body systems and is not limited to the issue under consideration. Questions about digestion, for instance, may be asked even if the presenting complaint is a skin rash or an orthopedic issue. TCVM involves assembling information into patterns which connect seemingly unrelated problems. For example, chronic otitis and chronic anal gland problems may have the same underlying cause. In addition, TCVM considers the patient's environment, a crucial factor in disease and diagnosis which is sometimes overlooked by Western medicine.

Hospice and Palliative Care

In his book *Being Mortal*, Dr. Atul Gawande describes a colleague's discussion with her father about the man's upcoming surgery for a spinal tumor. The colleague asked her father what sort of quality of life was most important to him, in case a decision regarding his care had to be made while he was under anesthesia.

Her father responded that he would be willing to stay alive if he were able to eat chocolate ice cream and watch football on television.

When Dr. Gawande's own father was diagnosed with a spinal tumor and faced increasing paralysis, he had different parameters for what he considered a good quality of life. The ability to watch television and eat his favorite food was *not* enough for him. Consequently, Dr. Gawande had different decision-making guidelines to follow while his father was undergoing spinal surgery (Gawande 2014, 183, 212).

These narratives relate to the quality-of-life conversations we frequently have in veterinary medicine. Hospice and palliative care are relatively new fields in veterinary medicine, and although our patients cannot communicate their preferences to us, we can learn from human NM. In addition, caring for sick and dying patients can result in a toll on the clinician's mental health, and the ability to practice reflection and self-compassion can be crucial to maintaining a good quality of life for the practitioner.

One Health

One Health looks at the big picture of the complex interactions and connections between human and animal health and that of the environment. Every day, veterinarians act as natural One Health practitioners, as the well-being of our patients is intertwined with that of their people. NM can help both illuminate and further these connections by examining them more closely.

An area only beginning to be explored is that of non-zoonotic conditions shared between animals and people who live together. In veterinary medicine, this often takes the form of a client disclosing they themselves have the same condition which the veterinarian is testing or treating their pet. One example is diabetes, and a study in the *BMJ* has found that owners of a dog with diabetes were more likely to develop type 2 diabetes themselves than owners of a dog without diabetes (Delicano et al. 2020). This sort of information is more likely to be shared in a narrative-style interaction with a practitioner than a purely clinical conversation. While the diabetes study findings could potentially result from something like a lifestyle or diet shared by human and pet, there are other possibilities. Another study found that dog owners shared more skin microbiota with their own dogs than with other dogs (Song et al. 2013).

Finally, human and veterinary medicine are far more alike than different, and a one-health/NM approach could allow clinicians to learn from one another's skills, approaches and experience, for optimal care of both humans and animals, and improved practitioner well-being.

Suggestions for Reflection and Discussion

- Were any of the related fields surprising to you?
- Which of the related fields do you find most important to the practice of veterinary medicine?
- Are there any fields you would add?
- Look up the Mindful Attention Awareness Scale online and answer the brief questionnaire to establish your own level of mindfulness. What areas might you need to work on?

The Veterinary Appointment

CHAPTER THREE

Before the Appointment

You're about to enter an exam room. What are you thinking about as your hand touches the door handle? Do you know who you are going to see, or will it be a surprise? How do you feel, physically? Emotionally? Do you need to use the bathroom? (Of course you do; go ahead and grab a bite of brownie on your way back.)

In a perfect world, every professional would enter the exam room calmly and with a clear mind, knowing something about, but not judging, the patient and client beforehand. While that is not always possible, this chapter examines how narrative medicine can make this a more likely scenario.

Key Points

- Consider the interaction you are about to have as the continuation of an ongoing narrative rather than an isolated episode.
- Reviewing your patient's record before entering the exam room may seem time-consuming; however, an increased awareness of the client and patient's history can enhance efficiency and set the client at ease.
- A mindful pause before an appointment can serve as a reminder to keep thoughts in the present, rather than the past or the future.
- Through narrative, we enter the unique "world" of our patient and client.
- A "beginner's mind" outlook can help us remain open to our client's narratives.

DOI: 10.1201/9781003126133-5

Why Read the Record First?

Consider the client and patient you are about to see. While your patient may be an enthusiastic Labrador who charges into the exam room looking for cookies, it is more likely the animal will be nervous. Quite often, an anxious patient is accompanied by an anxious client. Some clients are so agitated that the pet reacts to the owner's emotional state, compounding the stress level of both individuals.

There's been a recent focus on patient stress in veterinary medicine; one study demonstrated significant differences in several physiologic variables between measurements taken at home versus in the clinic setting (Bragg et al. January 15, 2015, Vol. 246, No. 2). The Fear Free® Initiative grew out of a desire to decrease stress and anxiety in companion animals during veterinary care and treatment; founder Dr. Marty Becker cautions against "focusing just on the pet's body, ignoring the mind" and emotions of the animal (Becker 2015). We do our best to calm our anxious patients with our soft touch and gentle voice, which can lead to decreased client anxiety. But can we also help calm a nervous patient by setting an anxious owner at ease?

A quick read-through of the patient's record can yield valuable information which can help the practitioner reassure the client before even approaching their animal. Although you may not have thought of Rex since his visit five months earlier, in the client's mind, today's visit is likely the continuation of her mental narrative, *Veterinary Visits with Rex*. By greeting the client with the statement, "I'm glad to see that Rex has been staying away from porcupines these days," you may be able to set the client at ease and affirm that you know her and Rex, even if you weren't the one to remove the quills.

Also check any notes the record contains regarding the personal history of the client and pet. A knowledge of details such as other household pets, family member's names, the fact that they moved to the area recently, or what the clients do for work can be helpful when the goal is to establish a connection and relationship. Starting the visit with a more personal remark than a comment on the weather does not mean you are going to spend the entire visit in mindless chitchat or that the client will think you want to be their new best friend. Rather, it is creating a positive rapport, so the client can feel comfortable discussing their animal with you.

- So, you're a dental hygienist! You'll have to tell me what you think of his teeth.
- I see you just moved, how is Fluffy adjusting to the new place?
- What do your kitties think of the new puppy?

A relaxed client can decrease your patient's stress level. In addition, an owner who is less anxious is more likely to recall and understand information from the visit, which could lead to increased compliance (Pickersgill and Owen 1992).

Reading the record connects you with the previous narrative of the patient. Imagine visiting a physician who greets you warmly when she enters the room but has no idea who you are or why you are there – even though you've visited the practice several times – and is unapologetic about her lack of information. Now imagine the same practitioner establishing a direct connection with you by initiating the conversation with an observation about a previous visit.

A scan through the record of a patient's last couple of appointments can provide information about their prior narrative. Even if nothing appears relevant, it is possible to link the animal's previous medical issues with the current visit by asking, *Does she still have a cough?* or *Is he still limping on that front leg?* Reviewing the record in more detail can give insight regarding a chronic problem such as otitis. A look at the dates of prior visits may help identify a problem which occurs seasonally. Other information can also be gleaned from patient records, including an understanding of how often the client visits (for instance, are there only sick visits listed, without wellness checks?) and the nature of any phone conversations with other doctors or staff. Even for a well-known patient, a review of the chart before the appointment could identify new information or help recall an overlooked aspect of the pet's history.

> Although you may not have thought of Rex since his visit five months earlier, in the client's mind, today's visit is likely the continuation of her mental narrative, "Veterinary Visits with Rex."

Prepare to Greet the Patient

Greeting the patient upon entering the exam room is another way to help a client relax. A positive comment about their animal can instantly change a client's focus from worry and concern to love and pride. Even if the patient is the ugliest, snarliest beast you've ever laid eyes on, try to find something positive to say.

- Hi there Lucky, it's so nice to meet you!
- Look at that gorgeous tail/those beautiful eyes/that lovely coat!
- I love that collar, it really suits him.
- Don't worry, Fluffy, you'll be home soon and then you can have a nice nap.

Consider Asking a Staff Member for Narrative Background

If patient information is sparse, consider checking with a staff member. The scheduling receptionist may have some insight based on a phone conversation or other contact with the client. If a technician or assistant did an intake, ask for their subjective assessment in addition to their objective summary. Did the client mention any concerns, such as a weight gain? Information such as the fact that an animal initially belonged to the client's child may or may not be noted in the chart but could have been relayed to the technician or receptionist.

Try to have a system in place for client records to note whether a client is a friend, neighbor, or relative of a staff member. If so, that person could be the source of valuable background information about both the animal and client.

But Who Has Time?

If examining the chart before entering the room is unfamiliar, it may seem like a luxury in terms of time. However, consider the ways you might gain time from reading the record first. By establishing a rapport with the client from the beginning of the appointment, communication may flow easily and quickly, while decreasing the client's and patient's anxiety. And a familiarity with the patient's history may save you time looking through the record later.

Mindfulness: Observe your Emotions

Narrative medicine (NM) takes some examples from the field of mindfulness, which is discussed in more detail in Chapters Two and Thirteen. On any particular day, a practitioner's emotional state may be a response to a client, a patient, the workplace environment, or any of a number of personal issues outside of work. While emotional responses can be challenging to control, the first step is to recognize they are present, without judging them.

Many clinic scenarios can elicit emotions that risk carrying over into the next appointment, including irritation, frustration, fatigue, and sadness. Issues with other staff members can cause tension, and the day might have been unusually busy. You may have just gotten off the phone with a difficult client, or delivered bad news to a favorite one.

The next appointment could also be a source of apprehension. A client's manner may cause irritation, especially if they are abrasive and/or demanding. Even if the client is new to you, they can induce stress by arriving late and throwing off the appointment schedule, or by bringing an additional pet "just for you to take a quick look at." In addition, fractious patients or challenging diagnoses can be causes of frustration. Finally, we all have lives outside of work. Lack of sleep, family or financial concerns, health issues, the weather, etc., all can affect our frame of mind.

In Chapter Thirteen, we will further examine how mindfulness can benefit practice, especially when combined with self-compassion.

The Mindful Pause

With all of this going on, how can you center yourself? Think of taking an intentional, mindful pause. Mindfulness reminds us to remain in the present, not in the past or the future. A focus on being mindful can increase awareness of where our brain wants to go instead, as it trains the brain to observe emotions and thoughts that arise without judgment. Once we are more aware of the feelings that come up, it becomes easier to set them aside and remain in the moment.

Here are some suggestions.

- Take a few deep breaths. Each breath provides an opportunity to release any bad feelings and renew. Breathe in fresh, new air. Try it with your eyes closed, if possible.
- When you wash your hands, try to focus on what you are doing in that moment. Feel the temperature of the water, your hands coming together. Don't think about something that just happened, or the next appointment. Consider that you are cleansing previous activity to make room for the next client and patient. When you are done, if you shake your hands, consider any residual concerns to be flying away with the droplets.
- Drink some water. Feel the liquid flowing down your throat, rehydrating and sustaining you.

Beginning the narrative on a good note can make the whole visit more efficient and comfortable for practitioner, patient, and client. While it may not be possible to *not* be annoyed, it may be possible to recognize any annoyance and attempt to set it aside. Otherwise, the client, patient, and staff members may sense your irritation, making it harder to interact successfully. A client may hold back information for fear of being judged. The patient may not allow as full of an exam. A staff member may not speak up about an important detail they want to bring to your attention.

Finally, mindfulness may be best considered as a continuum rather than an attainable goal; just noticing how you felt before, during, or after a visit is an enormous step toward a mindful practice. In addition, it's important to practice self-compassion, and remember that your best on one day may look different than your best on a different day.

Keep an Open Mind

Remember that the client may have a good explanation. If a client is late for my first appointment of the morning, I may worry about being backed up for the whole day, and I might become irritated. If the client explained that she was late due to a phone call with her child's oncologist, I would be far less annoyed. On the other hand, we cannot let clients take advantage of us, and firm policies can be essential. If a client is too late or chronically late, they may need to reschedule; if they bring an extra pet, they may have to reschedule or wait (for more on boundaries, see Chapter Thirteen).

> When possible, take a moment to focus on a deep breath while you wash your hands between appointments or take a drink of water, especially if you notice yourself feeling irritated, fatigued, or sad.

The Beginner's Mind

So, you've looked at the record and are about to enter the room. You've taken a deep breath and feel calm and focused despite the busy day. Now it's time to consider an important concept called the "beginner's mind." At the very beginning of his book *Zen Mind, Beginner's Mind*, Shunryu Suzuki writes, "In the beginner's mind there are many possibilities, but in the expert's there are few" (Suzuki 1970).

But who wants to be a beginner? Aren't we the expert? The client is paying us, surely that must mean something?

Let's unpack this.

A beginner's mind is not just an open mind, it is a mind which acknowledges that we do not know all the answers. It is a mind that is ready to learn and change. In veterinary medicine, it is literally possible to learn something new every day, and a beginner's mind is aware that some animals "didn't read the book" and may not fit into a classic diagnosis, or that the diagnosis is fluid and could change.

A beginner's mind stands in contrast with the expert's mind, which holds a narrow view, is resistant to change and prizes certainty.

The field of human NM values being comfortable with uncertainty, a quality also called having a "tolerance for ambiguity" or TFA (Gowda et al. 2018). There is a TFA scale used to evaluate medical students which has been adapted for veterinary students, as a low TFA has been linked to increased stress and possibly increased burnout (Hammond et al. 2017). In his book *Attending: Medicine, Mindfulness, and Humanity*, physician Ronald Epstein writes, "In medicine, feeling not-too-certain leads good clinicians to dig further, to explore the archaeology of each person's illness...mindful clinicians can feel confident while retaining some doubt." (Ronald Epstein 2017, 39,46).

Consider an experienced practitioner about to walk into an exam room containing a cat with a chronic skin problem. This doctor has treated hundreds, if not thousands, of cats with skin problems, and has treated this particular cat many times in the past. However, the practitioner has not treated *this* cat and *this* problem on *this* day. A beginner's mind is open to discovering something new, even if it is unlikely and unexpected.

Having a beginner's mind also means recognizing that the owner is the expert on their pet. Owners often identify subtle changes in their animal's habits, behaviors, and personalities and are usually correct about what is going on with them. If you cannot identify the problem with an animal, it can be helpful to ask the owner, "What do you think is going on?" Owner concerns should always be taken seriously and never dismissed out of hand.

As we seek to obtain a narrative which will illuminate our patient's condition, we rely on the client to bring forward information we need, information which may conflict with the data we receive from our examination or diagnostics. Faced with a lab report or radiograph that appears incompatible with life, it may be hard to believe the patient is still eating and playing. Yet while it is possible the client is in denial, most experienced practitioners have indeed seen many such cases. Also notable is the reverse situation: a patient clearly "ADR" with unremarkable test and physical exam results. In those cases, a wider view of the client's narrative may help identify the problem.

A beginner's mind is also valuable when we consider entering the narrative of another person, the world of our patient and client.

Prepare to Visit Another's Story

When we begin a story, we enter the world of the character (real or invented) in a book, television show, movie, or play, gauging the surroundings to gain context for the story. The effective practice of medicine involves entering the world of our patients in much the same way (Charon 2006, 9). The backdrop or home life of an animal patient can vary widely and is greatly affected by their human caretakers. The reality in the world of your patient and client may seem different from your reality; it may appear recognizable or unfamiliar, comfortable or awkward, surprising or predictable.

Imagine visiting a patient and client at home, a literal entry into their world. Here is where the patient eats and naps, the yard where they play, and the bed where they sleep. Details of the human–animal bond are also revealed – a cat's favorite sofa cushion, covered in grey fur; a dog bed by a fireplace; or a beautiful name plate over a horse's stall door. In that world, a "small amount of food" may prove to be a large overflowing bowl that is clearly not rationed despite the client claiming (and possibly believing) otherwise. A patient with a chronic cough may inhabit a home filled with an overwhelming odor of cigarette smoke; or, alternatively, a stifling aroma arising from numerous strongly scented candles and air fresheners. An equine veterinarian likely knows who maintains an immaculate barn and which patients reside in an area in need of a thorough cleaning.

In addition to the physical world of the patient, each animal guardian has a different worldview. This could also be thought of as the client's subjective reality, which contributes to their perspective. The client's worldview involves not only how they live their life, but also the nature of their relationship with their animal, the decisions they make regarding their animal, who else they consult with regarding their animal's care, and so on. Their animals also reside in this "world" and are subject to its tides and seasons, which may not make sense to outsiders. We as practitioners may not know or understand the underlying emotions and prior experiences contributing to a client's decisions and actions. Each has a different balance of structure and chaos, anxiety and calm, activity and rest. Worlds are messy and don't always make sense, and nearly all have blind spots (such as the overflowing food bowl) as well as pockets of dysfunction, denial, and skewed perspective, which may affect our patient's care. Bringing a beginner's mind to a consultation means we are open to learning about our patient's world.

Our client's narratives allow us to enter their world, so we may better understand the internal logic of the world inhabited by both patient and client (Murphy et al. 2018). A simple example is a patient with a painful tooth abscess and a client who refuses to allow her pet to undergo a dental procedure. Upon discussion with the client, you may learn that her childhood pet died under anesthesia while undergoing a dental procedure. In the client's world, animal dental procedures are not safe. With this knowledge, you can reassure her that while the risk is never zero, animal anesthesia is far safer now than it was decades ago due to preanesthetic blood tests, advances in anesthetics, and enhanced monitoring.

Case Story: *Entering the World of Patient and Client*

During one home visit, I conducted the exam of a large black Labrador on the owner's enclosed front porch. As I waited for the elderly owner to retrieve his checkbook from inside the house, I put my pen down on the end table next to me and noticed it rested on a road atlas from 1986. I looked closer to make sure I was reading it correctly. Then I wondered what new highways had been built since the atlas had last been used. I was unsurprised when the owner complained at the price of his dog's blood work. If his road atlas was stuck in the 1980s, his views on the cost of veterinary care likely were as well. To address his concerns, I focused my explanation on the value of the thyroid testing to his dog's health, and he agreed to the charges.

At another home visit in an immaculate townhouse, I was presented with a detailed chart which included everything my patient had consumed and eliminated since our last visit two weeks prior. This client was very detail-oriented and observant about her cat. When I gave her my recommendations, I knew they would be scrupulously followed to the best of her ability. I tried to be as specific as possible in my recommendations and explanations.

Another client, who lived alone with her dog, was continually ordering various processed foods from a home shopping network. At each visit, she generously insisted on sending me home with snacks from her latest delivery and always asked if a certain product was okay to feed her overweight dog. She described her dog as "picky" because she always had to tempt him to eat by topping his food with her most recent find. The client was in denial about her dog's weight issue and enjoyed sharing her food with him. I soon found that advising her not to feed the dog her snack foods was useless; instead, I concentrated on which ones would be the least detrimental to his health.

While some details may seem insignificant, having an image of a patient's home surroundings can help a practitioner respond to them as individuals and communicate more effectively. In a clinic setting, getting a sense of the patient's lived reality is more difficult, which is why it is important to gather what details we can through the client's narrative, the patient's chart, and conversations with staff members.

When You Know You'll Be Distracted

If you are worried about a patient "out back," waiting for a phone call, or need to check in with another client before they leave, you may want to let the client know before you get started.

"I may need to jump out of the room in a few minutes to check on a sick patient, but I wanted to get started with you and Coqui," you can inform the owner. This shows that you are thinking of their well-being, and lets them know the alternative to a potential interruption would be for their appointment to be further delayed.

Other options include setting a timer or tasking a staff member to alert you when necessary.

Case Story: *The Irritated Doctor*

I glanced at the schedule on the computer and frowned. How did *that* get booked? A sick 14-year-old dog, who hasn't been seen in over two years, had been newly scheduled into a 15-minute appointment slot.

I was annoyed at the receptionist for booking the time-pressured appointment and annoyed at the client, whom I supposed may have neglected her dog, before I even walked into the room.

The client, a frail elderly woman named Lillian, entered the room with a small, old mixed-breed dog. The little brown and white dog didn't appear to be in terribly bad shape, I noted, at least from across the room. As soon as the woman sat down, she began to cry.

"My husband just died last week. He was so sick for…for so long, and I spent all my time taking care of him," she confided. "I kept wanting to bring little Teddy in here, but I never seemed to have the time. Now I'm afraid I've neglected him."

My mood changed completely. I felt a surge of compassion for this woman, who had just lost her husband, and was now worried about her dog.

"It's okay," I assured her, "you're here now. I'm so sorry for the loss of your husband. That must have been so hard! Now, tell me, what's been going on with Teddy?"

I examined the little dog and drew some blood from him. He had some fluids administered, and I sent him home with some medication. The following day, I called Lillian from home to check in on Teddy and discuss his test results. Teddy had seemed better initially but now seemed to be losing his appetite again. I told Lillian that Teddy may need to visit the clinic sooner than the following week's recheck appointment with me, and as I only worked there two days per week, she would need to be seen by another of the clinic's doctors, perhaps the vet Teddy used to see regularly.

"Oh no," said Lillian, "I'd rather see you!"

I explained that we didn't want Teddy to have to wait if he wasn't feeling well. I felt a twinge of guilt thinking of my initial reaction to her appointment with Teddy. Ultimately, my irritation before seeing Lillian and Teddy may have negatively affected myself more than my client and patient.

Fortunately, Lillian described her situation as soon as I entered the room; I likely would have felt even worse had it come to light later in the encounter. It was a good reminder for me to not judge a client's situation and to enter the room with an open mind, letting go of any assumptions and biases which had occurred to me upon seeing the appointment on the schedule.

Suggestions for Reflection and Discussion

- How do you begin appointments? Try to notice your state of mind before you enter the room, without judging.
- Consider how you might take a mindful pause before entering an exam room.
- How often do you read the previous record's notes before seeing a patient? Has it been helpful?
- Do you ever speak to staff members about a patient before stepping into the room?
- Think of some examples of a "beginner's mind" and an "expert mind."
- Describe the world view of one of your more eccentric clients (or relatives).

CHAPTER FOUR

Obtaining a History

What happens when you walk into an exam room or a barn and encounter your patient and their caretaker(s)? How can we obtain a history that includes a full picture of the life of our patient? If we view our patient's history as a story, it can be a road toward a greater understanding of our patient's needs and effective treatment.

Key Points

- A chronological viewpoint fits better in two dimensions, but real life is three-dimensional; Narrative Medicine (NM) can help us move beyond a chronological understanding of a patient's history.
- NM involves guiding the conversation according to what the client is saying in real time, with the goal of picking up on the client's narrative to determine what questions to ask next.
- Techniques to invite and recognize narratives include close listening, nonverbal communication, the opening question, considering point of view, and narrative questioning.
- "Problems in Parentheses" are the client's underlying concerns that can affect their decisions about their pet.

What Is a History?

Consider the history of a famous individual such as Ernest Hemingway or Marie Curie. To gain an understanding of the person, it would be necessary to understand the time and place in which he or she lived, as well as their words and deeds.

DOI: 10.1201/9781003126133-6

How much would you learn about the person from reading a Wikipedia entry compared to reading an in-depth biography or watching a compelling documentary? The Wikipedia entry is likely a list of data points, telling a two-dimensional story. A biography or documentary should give context and insight to the story, as things don't necessarily happen in a linear fashion. Seeing the history as a story helps "bring the past alive," allowing us to view the history in a three-dimensional manner.

Considering a patient's history as a story fits well with current descriptions of obtaining a medical history, such as the use of open-ended questions favored by the Calgary-Cambridge guide (Kurtz and Silverman 2005).

Inviting and Recognizing Narratives

To enter our patient's world, we need to listen to the narrative of their caretaker. But how do you invite someone to tell you a story? The goal is to make it as easy as possible for the client to tell you the patient's story, which is naturally part of their own story.

Along with creating a positive environment for our client to relate a narrative, we must also be able to recognize narratives when we see them.

In this chapter, we explore:

- Close listening
- Nonverbal communication
- The opening question
- Point of view
- Narrative and circular questioning
- Problems in Parentheses

Close Listening: Seeking Out the Story

"We cannot learn what we must learn about and from patients by asking everyone the same set of questions," writes Dr. Rita Charon. "Instead, we health professionals have to equip ourselves with radically more flexible and creative skills." (Charon 2006, 187). One of the skills Dr. Charon describes is "close listening," and she explains how we need to listen "for" stories and not just listen "to" them; we need to seek out our patients' stories. Narratives tend to be messy and nonlinear, and don't fit neatly into the outlines many of us have been taught to use. As tempting as it may be to redirect the client when they go "off topic" and talk about something other than the specific question you've asked, you may miss the narrative. Consider the case of a vomiting cat. A practitioner could spend quite some time interviewing the client about the duration and frequency of vomiting, amount and composition of vomitus, and relationship to eating while taking copious notes. Yet a confession from a client that they are missing a sewing needle might have the cat in question heading swiftly toward the x-ray table.

Nonverbal Communication

An essential part of inviting a story is to assure the teller you are listening, and nonverbal language is likely something both listener and teller rely upon more than we realize. In veterinary medicine, we routinely observe nonverbal cues from our clients, our patients, and their interactions with one another. We are skilled at interpreting nonverbal language from our patients. But what about the clues from our clients? And how might we come across ourselves?

An observational study that examined nonverbal communication between physicians and patients found that doctors who used gestures and leaned slightly toward their patients received higher ratings from them. Nonverbal cutoffs at the end of the appointment, such as looking away from the patient, earned low ratings from patients (Little et al. 2015).

The best model for examining nonverbal communication I have found comes from an unlikely source: a stop-motion animation television series by the creators of Wallace and Gromit called Shaun the Sheep. In addition to being an enjoyable show for all ages, each 7-minute episode is an excellent study of just how effective nonverbal communication can be.

Unlike Wallace and Gromit, no language is spoken in Shaun the Sheep. The characters – the farmer, his dog, several sheep (including the title character), assorted pigs, chickens, and other animals as well as the occasional visiting human – communicate nonverbally and with occasional grunts or whistles. Despite this limitation, the characters understand each other quite well; it is not a show where plot lines commonly involve miscommunication. Even within the limits of Claymation, characters communicate clearly and effectively using a tilt of the head, a shrug of the shoulders, a widening of the eyes, a gesture, or a glance. After watching a couple of episodes, spoken language seems superfluous.

Nonverbal cues are especially important when the goal is for a client to comfortably relate a narrative. The client should receive the message that they have your full attention; even if you are examining the animal or jotting notes, be sure to speak to and look at the client. However, it is not enough to simply make eye contact and let the client speak. The listening must be done closely and authentically to discover the narrative. Consider the nonverbal cues you might use if a close friend or relative is about to tell a story you are anxious to hear. Your posture, gestures, and facial expressions would communicate interest and an intent to listen closely. Now imagine the story is somewhat awkward, and your loved one is hesitant to continue. Your nonverbal communication would want to indicate that it is safe to continue because you are listening openly and nonjudgmentally.

Observing the Human–Animal Bond

Part of the nonverbal communication we observe during an appointment is the interaction between patient and client. Is the animal calmed by the owner's voice? What is the owner's expression when she looks at her pet: is it worry, affection, frustration? Is the dog a family pet, a hunting dog, a single person's companion? As we explore further in Chapter Seven, The Connection Triangle, human and pet are bonded, and their narratives are intertwined. The nature of their relationship provides context and is essential to understanding the patient's story.

Close Listening over the Phone: Attending to the Voice

Sometimes, we need to have important conversations with clients over the phone. This was especially the case during the pandemic, as many clinics did not allow clients to enter the building. Conversations unfolded over the phone or in a busy parking lot. During nonpandemic times, we also speak to clients on the phone, and even deliver bad news and have important euthanasia or quality-of-life discussions. Often, though, we have recently seen them in the office and are following up with test results or answering a client's question. If we already know the patient and client and understand their relationship, we can use the knowledge obtained in previous interactions to inform our understanding of a telephone interaction.

During telephone conversations, we can utilize many of the same skills we practice when the client is in front of us, with the obvious exception of nonverbal communication. Phone calls are an excellent time to practice close listening. Without the distraction of visual stimuli and without the patient present, we can fully focus on the nuances of the client's voice, such as any pauses or hesitation, and emphasis placed on certain words or phrases. Important phone conversations are best handled in a quiet area, without the distraction of barking dogs or interruptions from coworkers.

Close Watching over Telemedicine: Attending to the Surroundings

Telemedicine use is increasing, and there are some benefits in NM terms. One advantage is that we are allowed a rare view inside the patient and client's home. We also see the patient in what is likely their most relaxed surroundings, so it's an opportunity to encounter and evaluate a side of them we might not see at the clinic or even during a home visit. If the client is using a mobile device, the clinician can ask to see where the patient eats and sleeps. When dietary issues are evaluated in the home, there can be a surprising contrast between the amount a client claims to feed and the amount of food in the bowl(s) (and the "one cup" they use to measure may turn out to be a large Solo brand cup). We may also be able to identify and assist clients with behavioral issues like temperament mismatch problems, such as the timid animal in the chaotic household, which the client may not realize is chaotic because to them, it is normal. Suggestions could include having a quiet out-of-the-way corner or room for the animal to retreat to and adding a pheromone diffuser.

The Opening Question

How do you begin a conversation with a client after greeting them? The Calgary-Cambridge guide calls this the "opening question" (Kurtz and Silverman 2005). You want to know why the client and patient are there today, which is usually written on the record, but could be different from what you are assuming or have been informed by a technician. By inviting a story, you can also see what the client emphasizes, which can be a clue to an underlying problem, especially in the common case of the ADR patient.[1] For instance, if the client emphasizes that the animal has appeared to be in pain, that is important information, especially if the patient does not appear painful to you at the time.

The goal of the "opening question" from a NM perspective is to invite the client to tell the patient's *story*, rather than recite a disjointed litany of facts and details. When the facts are related as part of a story, the information is often more accessible, and the client more likely to feel their issues have been heard.

There is no one "right" opening question. Think about how you usually start a conversation with a client. Many of us probably have our own favorites; we

---

1 ADR stands for "Ain't Doin' Right, a reference to the writings of Alf Wight as James Herriott, when farmers would tell him that their cow just *ain't doin right*. It has become a commonly used term for a patient that is just not themselves with vague symptoms.

may even use them automatically, out of habit. Our level of formality may vary depending upon how well we know the client. Common opening questions are:

- "What brings you here today?"
- "So, I hear Fluffy isn't feeling well?"
- "What's been going on with Fluffy?"
- "How has Fluffy been lately?"

My personal go-to question is, "When did you notice a problem?" or "When did you first notice a problem?" This is my attempt to invite a story in chronological terms and have the client begin the story at the beginning of the issue.

> The goal of the "opening question" from a NM perspective is to invite the client to tell the patient's story, rather than recite a disjointed litany of facts and details.

Point of View – Who Is Narrating?

The concept of "point of view" is one that is easy to examine from a literature or narrative standpoint: who is telling the story? (Charon 2006, 112). If we are considering our patient's story, the client is the narrator. How reliable are they? Do they contradict themselves? These are the same questions that come up when we open a book or watch a movie and begin a story. What questions do we have; what has been left out of the story for us to discover?

How does a storyteller frame the story? Think about a client's description of their animal as a photograph they are cropping. What do they notice, and what do they emphasize? What do they *not* notice or describe? (Charon 2006, 114–116)

Point of view is an entryway to the client's world view. In veterinary medicine, the world view of one guardian of an animal may not be the same as another's; for instance, one person may be more concerned about a new lump on their pet because they are naturally anxious and had a childhood pet who died of cancer. The other may have a less anxious nature and never had a pet who had cancer. Their world views differ, and your patient lives with both; how does this affect the animal? Another example of differing world views can be observed when a couple asks you to settle a bet about their animal (often involving whether the pet is overweight or not). Although it can be uncomfortable to be in the middle of a family argument, it is a good way to get a sense of the world views of the owners.

Consider who is telling the story of this animal and what their relationship is to the pet and to the rest of the household. Sometimes, the person presenting the animal is not the primary caretaker. Even if they are the official caretaker, someone else may feed, exercise, or clean the litter box. An awareness of what is *not* being told can help determine what questions to ask.

Guiding the Conversation – What about the Talkative Client?

Many practitioners worry that allowing the client free rein to tell their story will result in a long-winded account of everything from the day's weather and traffic to the client's childhood pets. Yet allowing the client to tell a story does not mean that you are not guiding the conversation. Ideally, the conversation will flow smoothly although we know that doesn't always happen and every practice has its notably long-winded clients. NM involves guiding the conversation according to what the client is saying in real time, with the goal of picking up on the client's narrative to determine what questions to ask next. Utilizing NM techniques may even shorten consultation times, as a focused approach can allow the practitioner to understand the nature of the issue more quickly than cycling through a long checklist of questions.

Narrative and Circular Questioning

According to a veterinary study on diet history questioning, the open-ended question, "Tell me…" yielded more information than the questions, "What kind of food…" and "What kind of foods…" (Coe et al. 2020). This makes sense because "Tell me…" is an invitation to tell a story. By saying "Tell me…," you are giving the client an open invitation to speak on a topic. Again, it is important to see what the client emphasizes, because that can give you clues to both the patient's problem and the world of the client and patient.

- Tell me what happened.
- Tell me more about ….
- Tell me what *you* think (is going on, the problem is, happened, etc.)

Here are some examples of narrative questioning:

Client: It was when Rocky had one of his episodes...
Doctor: Can you tell me about his episodes?
Client: Zoey had a bad day yesterday.
Doctor: What is a bad day like for Zoey?
Client: He just hasn't been himself.
Doctor: What makes you say that? Or, What have you noticed that's different?

It is important to adapt your questions to the unfolding conversation rather than follow a set list you may hold in your mind (Launer 2018, 43). This also helps the conversation feel more relaxed, and the client may feel more comfortable sharing information than if subjected to a previously curated rapid-fire list of questions, which offers little or no opportunity to relay their own narrative.

To understand the narrative of our patient, we need to expand upon the traditional linear questioning model to interview our patient's caretakers. The linear model objective is to determine a precise chronological timeline of events, which can be valuable. Yet although the linear model may make the most sense in a two-dimensional setting, such as an x and y graph, the body itself exists in a three-dimensional state of multiple simultaneous processes and interactions; consider the numerous feedback loops and cascades vital to survival (Launer 2002, 26). Relevant information may not fit neatly into the linear model, and animal caretakers sometimes struggle to describe their concerns within a linear framework, especially when they are stressed. A broader view of history-taking can help us better understand our clients, and ultimately our patients. While this is termed circular questioning, it may also be understood as contextual questioning, putting the concerns of the client into context.

Allowing the client to speak uninterrupted is another important consideration. Even if they seem to be off on a tangent, pay attention to where their story is going, as they may have a reason for bringing up a certain topic. It may involve a previous animal; many clients have conflicting feelings about previous pets and how they managed their care, and these emotions and memories could affect their current decision making.

If You Get Stuck, Take it Back to the Patient

Sometimes it's hard to connect with a client, especially one who is frustrated, irritable, or anxious. Even if their mood has nothing to do with you or their animal's condition, it can make communication difficult. A good way to handle this is to turn the topic of conversation to something complimentary about the patient.

This can help the client to relax and refocus, as most people love to hear wonderful things said about their pet.

- Look at her beautiful shiny coat; it's so soft. Do you brush her?
- How did he get his name? It really suits him.
- What beautiful expressive eyes she has!
- I love the way he folds his paws, that's adorable.

After a short conversation about how their pet is special, try going back to what you were discussing before, or use it as an opportunity to steer the conversation in a different direction.

Case Story: *The Dog with Osteosarcoma and the Angry Client*[2]

Nala was a new patient at the clinic, in for a holistic consult. She was a sweet 9-year-old boxer mix owned by a young couple. The dog was non-weight-bearing on her left front leg and had just been diagnosed with osteosarcoma at another veterinary clinic.

Nala's female owner was very pleasant, but her male owner was a different story. He sat on the bench in the exam room, his arms folded, exuding anger. He didn't make eye contact as he threw out his questions. *Why can't they just remove the tumor? Why would they have to amputate the whole leg?* The woman calmly explained that they couldn't afford surgery anyway. The couple's two young daughters played with a phone as I examined Nala and carefully answered the man's questions, explaining the serious nature of the disease.

I couldn't seem to connect with the male owner, so I considered asking a question I often ask on holistic consults, with the goal of trying to get a wide-angle view of the animal's medical history. In this case, however, I was attempting to prompt a narrative from the client.

"Have you had Nala since she was a puppy?" I asked casually, as my hands palpated her lymph nodes.

"*He* has," responded the woman, tilting her head toward her husband.

Ah.

I thought back to my own first dog, and how she'd been my buddy when I was single. We'd done everything together, and we had made a great team. She had

---

2 This case discussion is taken from an article by the author in a DVM360 article in 2017 entitled *Understand Your Veterinary Client's Narrative*.

been a constant presence through many changes in my life. Perhaps this man felt the same way about Nala.

The remainder of the appointment was still sad and painful, yet I felt that I had gained a greater understanding of this angry man. It helped me communicate with him and avoid overreacting to his strong emotions. Anger, I knew, was one of the five stages of grief identified by Dr. Elisabeth Kubler-Ross in her landmark book, *On Death on Dying* (Kubler-Ross 1969); I realized that I should not take his anger personally as it was in fact a sign of his grief over Nala's diagnosis.

To speak with him, I stayed crouched on the floor with Nala, in an unthreatening position. I knew the man likely also felt insecure because he did not understand what was happening to his dog. I explained why the tumor could not be removed without amputating the leg. I told him his beloved dog had a bad disease that she did not deserve, and it was not due to anything he had done, or not done. I dispensed some supplements but explained that they were not going to cure his dog. We discussed pain management and what to expect as the disease progressed. When they left, the man was much calmer.

When I later discussed the visit with a colleague, she said, "So, for that man, the dog may have represented his youth and freedom." The lives of our pets span certain time periods of our lives, and the death of a pet may seem like the end of an era. Understanding what a pet may represent to a person, in addition to the human–animal bond they share, can be helpful. That dog was the man's first responsibility before his children were born. While I did not get to witness obvious evidence of their human–animal bond itself, the strength of it was evident by his behavior.

Some people come in with a sick animal and are very forthcoming about their relationship with their pet, their current life circumstances, the involvement of other family members, and how it all ties together. With others, figuring out these things may take some work.

Recognizing Problems in Parentheses

The term Problems in Parentheses was inspired by the writings of my grandfather, Maurice Fine, a physician who practiced in Johannesburg, South Africa. My grandfather was a member of his community, whether doing home visits or seeing patients in his small office. Although he died in 1991, during my final year of veterinary school, my father recently discovered a folder tucked away in an old briefcase that contained some of his writings.

To keep a good balance between the scientific and the human – the interplay – this is what makes a doctor what he is, my grandfather had written.

In the old days, many a person found comfort in discussing her problems with her family doctor, who was often of real assistance, who listened to her story, and who put things in their proper perspective. Her backache was no more than a mild lumbago – no slipped disc in those days – and meanwhile, the real reason for her visit to the doctor was mentioned, and dealt with, almost in parentheses.

I knew exactly what my grandfather meant. It's when someone calls because their dog is sick, but their real concern has to do with the animal's quality of life. It's a person asking what you would do if it were your animal, when what they really want is reassurance that they are doing the right thing.

Problems in Parentheses are the issues that people find difficult to discuss yet may have a profound effect on both the client and patient. In veterinary medicine, they often involve our client's underlying emotions of fear, guilt, anxiety, sadness, confusion, or frustration regarding their animal friend, their concerns about their own ability to make decisions and adequately care for them, and their dread of losing them.

Dr. Charon discusses the importance of fully listening and responding to the "patient's narrative questions: 'What is wrong with me?' 'Why did this happen to me?' and 'What will become of me?'" (Charon 2001). In veterinary medicine, these questions can be understood as,

- "What is wrong with my animal?"
- "Why did this happen to us?"
- "What will become of us?"

Although the questions could perhaps be more directly translated by replacing "us" with "my animal," the client may perceive that the animal's issue is happening to them, as it affects them profoundly; it is happening to a household member for whom they are a caretaker.

To detect Problems in Parentheses, try to notice whether there is an underlying emotional current coming from the client. In the previous story, Nala's male owner's Problems in Parentheses – anger, confusion, and frustration – were overwhelming to everyone in the room. However, they are typically more subtle. In the example about the dog in need of a dental procedure from Chapter Three, the Problem in Parentheses was the client's anxiety about anesthesia.

The following story provides another example of a Problem in Parentheses.

Case Story: *Salmon's Story,* by Dr. Lauren Bookbinder

Salmon was an upper-level Saddlebred who presented for severe, acute colic. His pain was uncontrollable, and surgical exploration immediately recommended. At surgery, Salmon had a torsion of his large colon, which was corrected. He recovered uneventfully for about 18 hours and then began to colic severely. I suspected that he had either retwisted his colon or his colon was becoming necrotic.

His owner Kathy, a middle-aged woman who had horses all her life, said, "I waited my whole life for this horse. If there is any chance, take him back to surgery." At surgery, Salmon's colon was both retwisted and devitalized. Radical colon resection was the only chance he had, and it was slim at best.

"If there is a chance, take it." she said.

"Well, there is always a *chance*. But his prognosis is grave." I said, imaging the very long road ahead of this horse even if he could beat the odds.

We proceeded with surgery.

Salmon had a few OK days of recovery and then became very, very sick; he had developed a septic abdomen. His owner visited every day for a week of intensive supportive care, brushing him, and talking to me about their show career. She had only had him a few years and they had a lot of success in that short time. I really felt for her, but also really didn't get it. He was suffering, and she kept talking about how much she loved him, how long she had waited for him, and giving him a chance.

I felt myself starting to judge her.

"If she really loved him, she would let him go."

"Does she just want to show him again and win more classes? Sell him for lots of money? How selfish!"

And then, during one of her visits, I learned what Salmon really meant to Kathy. About 6 months prior, at their big national final show of the season, Kathy developed a cardiac arrhythmia while riding Salmon in a show class. Immediately after finishing the class, Kathy lost consciousness and was rushed to the hospital. She was transferred to an intensive cardiac unit for emergency ablation of her arrhythmia. She very nearly died, and believed that Salmon protected her and took care of her during their ride when the arrhythmia developed. He wasn't her pet or her show horse; he was truly her partner. Asking her to let go of him was like asking her to let go of her husband. After about a week of hospitalization, Salmon's role as partner and protector ever-so-slightly shifted back toward pet, and Kathy was able to let him go peacefully (Lauren Bookbinder 2021).

In the above story, the client Kathy felt as though she needed to go to extraordinary lengths to save Salmon's life because she felt that he had saved her life; she felt she owed him a debt beyond that of a beloved pet and companion.

The story is also notable for Dr. Bookbinder's mindful realization that she was beginning to judge the client. This realization helped Dr. Bookbinder to ask herself why Kathy would go to such extreme lengths to keep Salmon alive. The clinician's refusal to blindly judge was rewarded by the owner trusting her enough to reveal the truth about her relationship with her horse.

> To keep a good balance between the scientific and the human – the interplay –
> this is what makes a doctor what he is.
>
> Maurice Fine, MD, the author's grandfather

The Problem with Drop-Offs

Imagine a sick child dropped off at the pediatrician's office, perhaps with a scrawled, handwritten note detailing vomiting and a lack of appetite. As you are not the child's regular doctor, you need to examine a child you are not familiar with, not knowing whether the child's behavior at the office could be considered normal for him; whether he is typically stoic or anxious, high energy or calm. You also don't know the parents, so you don't have an understanding of the child's home life and background. You track down the receptionist who admitted the child, as well as the person who took the initial phone call, to try and get an idea of what could be going on. You may have little information on changes in diet and home surroundings. If your physical exam findings are unremarkable, you'll have to rely on performing some blood tests and/or radiographs to try to figure out a diagnosis. Once you arrive at a conclusion, you'll have to guess at whether the parents could medicate the child at home. Should you prescribe liquid? Chewable pills? Should you recommend a diet change? What does the child normally eat? Of course, you try to reach the parents on the phone. After leaving a detailed message on the first phone number the mother left, you finally reach her at the second number and go over your findings and treatment plan at length. You hang up only to be told by a receptionist that the child's anxious father is on hold on another line, waiting for an update. So, of course, you speak to him as well.

Ultimately, you will have spent far more time on this patient than a regular office appointment, and despite your best efforts, the patient's care could arguably be considered suboptimal.

Suggestions for Reflection and Discussion

- Notice how you begin conversations with clients. What kind of Opening Questions do you use? Do they make it easy for the client to tell a story?
- Watch a couple of episodes of "Shaun the Sheep" on YouTube (episodes are

only 7 minutes long). A couple of good ones are "Fossil" and "The Genie."
Are you surprised by how much of communication can be nonverbal?
- Think of a client with a sick animal you spoke to recently. How would you describe the person's emotional state? Do you think they have a Problem in Parentheses?
- How does your practice handle drop-offs?

CHAPTER FIVE

Making a Plan

Now you are part way through the visit with a client and patient. You've gotten a history, examined your patient, and are ready for the next step in the appointment.

It's time to make a plan.

Key Points

- The goal is to reach a new narrative together with your client, in partnership.
- It is important to work within the client's world view, even if you don't like the world and are glad you don't live there!
- Problems in Parenthesis are underlying emotional issues that should be addressed, often through validation.
- Self-disclosure can help us connect to clients as fellow pet owners and not only as veterinarians and staff. Clients may also benefit from hearing other people's narratives.

Reaching a New Narrative

The idea is simple: a client arrives with a narrative about their pet, and they leave with a new narrative. The new narrative is not handed to them like a prescription from their doctor, *it is cocreated with the practitioner* (Launer 2002, 29–30). Although the practitioner may have some initial ideas about a narrative they would like to establish, the new narrative cannot be imposed; it must be crafted during a conversation with the patient's caretaker. The result is truly individualized

DOI: 10.1201/9781003126133-7

medicine, as each new narrative is unique to that practitioner, that patient, and that caretaker.

The new narrative might involve reassurance to a conflicted person, reflecting a Problem in Parentheses of anxiety and self-doubt: *Am I doing the best for my friend?*

The doctor may respond, *I think you are doing a great job! I know it's not easy with all her issues. Let's see how she does on the new diet, and here is the medication we spoke about. I'll see you again next week.*

The case study from the previous chapter involved an angry client and his dog, Nala, with osteosarcoma. The client didn't fully understand what he was told by another doctor and was understandably distraught to have received a terminal diagnosis for his lovely and otherwise healthy dog. As we spoke, his emotional intensity decreased because he was able to understand the situation better and I directly addressed the source of his pain: the unfairness of the diagnosis. The client's initial narrative was some version of *Why can't you help Nala?* Together, we created a new narrative: *Nala has a bad disease, which is both greatly unfair and no one's fault, and although we can try to help there is not much we can do.*

Consider the Client's World View, Including Preconceived Ideas

As evidenced in the above story, not everyone understands the explanations we give, even if we do our best to clarify them for laypeople. Although it might seem obvious to us that a tumor in a bone would require an amputation to remove it, some clients will not realize or understand this. Dr. Annie Wayne, Assistant Professor at Cummings School of Veterinary Medicine at Tufts University, also recommends we take seriously our advice to other veterinarians and staff members about their own pets, and not assume they have the same information and understanding of their pet's condition that we may have.

A client's world view might cause them to interpret our explanations or recommendations in ways we do not anticipate. Additionally, people often have preconceived ideas based on past experiences, misunderstandings, or information obtained online. They may have personal biases, for instance, against treatments such as chemotherapy or steroids, and surgeries such as an amputation or enucleation. World views can arise from a client's family; perhaps they were raised to believe cats should never stay indoors, a pet rabbit would have no need for a veterinarian, or animals should be euthanized when first diagnosed with a serious illness.

Cancer and chemotherapy are likely the words that most often cause clients to recoil. If you say the word "cancer" to some people, you may as well have invited the Grim Reaper into the exam room and asked him to settle in for a chat. Some clients will be so distressed they won't even register subsequent explanations regarding "benign" versus "malignant," biopsy reports, or other related topics.

The word "chemo" is almost as bad, and in many people's minds, it is equivalent to the word "suffering." Some will immediately think of a friend or relative who has experienced chemotherapy – or as it's often phrased, has *gone through* chemotherapy – or they may have experienced it themselves. It is important to discuss the fact that there are many different chemotherapy protocols, as "chemo" is often talked about as one thing, and clients might mistakenly assume there is only one type of chemo drug or protocol. In addition, without the anxiety that typically surrounds people receiving chemotherapy, animals often respond differently. Finally, there are many medications as well as treatments such as acupuncture that can help alleviate side effects such as decreased appetite and nausea.

A phrase often repeated by clients after a serious diagnosis is that they "don't want to put him through" a test, procedure, or even a referral. While this may, indeed, be the best decision for their animal (for example, someone might reasonably decide to not pursue radiation therapy for a cat who becomes extremely stressed during car rides and veterinary visits), it can also represent a misunderstanding on their part. If someone doesn't understand what an ultrasound involves, they may believe anesthesia is required or their pet will be in pain during the procedure. It is important to confirm that the client is basing decisions on accurate and updated information, not about something that happened to their childhood pet, or the experiences of their neighbor or online friend whose dog had cancer, or their imagination. The "don't want to put him through" phrase is also sometimes used by clients to justify something they cannot afford. If you believe the patient could benefit from the treatment, test, or procedure you are discussing, it is worth unpacking the phrase with the client to determine their reasoning.

Addressing Problems in Parentheses

Problems in Parentheses may seem unnecessary or at best a low priority to address, yet these discussions can make an enormous difference to the client as well as your relationship with them. And anything affecting the animal's primary caretaker can relate directly to our animal patient. If the client is feeling anxious about her ability to care for her pet, the animal will pick up on the anxiety. If a client is frustrated about his cat's continued medical issue, he might elect euthanasia rather than continuing to treat. A client confused about their pet's diagnosis could ignore treatment recommendations.

Negative emotional experiences can also convince an individual to not obtain another pet in the future (see the excerpt of *The Friend* by Sigrid Nunez in

Chapter Eight), depriving another animal of a loving home, the person of an animal friend, and your practice of a valued client.

To address Problems in Parentheses, we must first recognize there is an issue. Consider the example in the previous chapter about the dog with a tooth abscess. Once we have realized the client is anxious about anesthesia due to an experience with a previous pet, we can reassure her that things have changed and emphasize that her pet is suffering without the procedure.

Simply acknowledging the client's concerns and validating the difficulties of caring for an ill animal can be immensely helpful. Responding to a Problem in Parentheses is often as straightforward as reassuring a client that they are doing the best they can, you agree with their decision(s), or the problem with their animal is not their fault. Alternatively, it may require a discussion regarding causation of disease, or the risks and benefits of treatment options. It may involve a reflection (mirroring) of their emotions, especially if a client is frustrated: simply saying you understand their frustration can be helpful as it validates their concerns, allowing them to feel understood. Sharing that it is common for pet owners to feel a certain way under similar circumstances, or that you have seen similar responses from other clients (more on that soon), can make a client feel as though they are not alone and their reactions are "normal" and understandable.

Addressing Problems in Parentheses is different for each situation, but it is an important part of veterinary practice.

A client's world view might cause them to interpret our explanations or recommendations in ways we do not anticipate. Additionally, people often have preconceived ideas based on past experiences, misunderstandings, or information obtained online.

Case Story from Human Narrative Medicine: *A Child with Eczema*

This case study is excerpted from a book by John Launer. Although it does not involve an animal patient, the situation is a common one for small animal veterinary practitioners and involves the validation of a Problem in Parentheses.

Mr. and Mrs. J. are a couple whose son Jake, age 2, has severe atopic eczema. Jake's parents say they are frantic at their inability to stop Jake scratching, and also because of sleep deprivation.

Their nurse practitioner knows there is evidence that they should be giving

Jake daily baths, using copious amounts of skin emollients, and topical steroids in limited quantities. When she proposes this, however, their response is one of despondency. They cannot imagine fitting the regime of meticulous skin care into their lives, especially as they also have a 4-year-old and a new baby. They have also heard awful things about steroids. They say they would like to see a specialist for allergy tests.

Commentary: The tension here between narrative and evidence may arise because the parents' original narrative was not in fact about Jake's eczema but about their own helplessness and exhaustion. The way to reach a convergence of stories might be for the nurse to set aside for a moment her own chosen evidence-based narrative of treating Jake's skin and to concentrate instead on their unmanageable feelings.

For example, she might offer Mr. and Mrs. J. an alternative narrative that described eczema as "the itching disease". She might also reassure them that parental desperation with eczema is extremely common, and might be especially heightened for parents with two other under-fives. This might lessen their sense of ineffectiveness and give them a chance to open up a story about taking more control of Jake's condition. If this happens, they may be more likely to heed her advice – or she may be more likely to agree to a referral as something that the parents need to take their own story forwards.

(Launer 2002, 61–62)

Responding to a Problem in Parentheses is often as simple as reassuring a client that they are doing the best they can, you agree with their decision(s), or the problem with their animal is not their fault.

Healing through Life Experience and Attention

In the words of Rachel Naomi Remen, founder of The Healer's Art program used for both medical and veterinary students, "We cure with our expertise but we heal with our life experience and our attention." (Remen 2016)

Remen lists two different components to healing, and both are individualized. Note that she refers not to our *clinical* experience but to our *life* experience, which can help us interpret our practice experience and integrate it with our ability to connect with the pet owner. Our "life experience" is uniquely our own; we each have a unique history which has helped shape us and naturally affects our work.

Different practitioners also have different practice styles. Some clinicians are soft-spoken and some are more forceful; some take their time and others are more brusque. Some practitioners are optimists and some are pessimists. We've also had different instructors at different schools with different philosophies. Clients' personalities vary too, and people will gravitate toward doctors with whose practice styles they feel most comfortable. There is no such thing as an "ideal" life experience or a "correct" practice style. We each connect with clients in our own, unique way.

Remen also uses the word "attention." Attention is an important part of narrative medicine and is discussed in Chapter One's section on Dr. Rita Charon's work on Attention, Representation, Affiliation, as well as Chapter Two's section on Mindfulness. Attention is the energy and the part of ourselves we give to the interaction. By bringing our attention to the client to cocreate a plan for our patient, we forge a unique connection.

Case Story: *Euthanasia with a Different Doctor*

One of my coworkers, Dr. Mulcahy, was presented a dog for euthanasia. The dog was old and ill, and the clients were not ambivalent about the euthanasia decision. However, the people were upset because their regular veterinarian at the practice, whom they had been working closely with, was away on vacation and the dog's condition was such that they were unable to wait for her return. The clients felt things were not as they should have been. Their sadness and unease about the situation made the already painful appointment even harder for them.

Dr. Mulcahy flipped through the dog's chart and noticed her own handwriting at the very beginning of the record, on the dog's first visit to the clinic as a puppy. She then offered the clients a new narrative: she was the very first one to see the dog at the clinic, and she would also be the last, bookending the dog's life. The clients gladly embraced the new narrative and were able to let go of the sense that their dog's passing was premature and ill-timed.

In this story, the doctor gave the grieving caretakers the gift of feeling as though their dog's euthanasia was perfectly timed and "meant to be." By paying close attention and not taking the situation personally, she was able to provide the clients with what they really needed at that moment: a way to accept the other doctor's absence. As we explore further in Chapter Eight, Grief, Guilt, and Shame, negative experiences around euthanasia and death are particularly significant, and can lead to long-lasting negative and dysfunctional narratives for the client, affecting subsequent pets.

Supporting the Human–Animal Bond

In Chapter Seven, the Connection Triangle, we will explore the human–animal bond and its importance in the daily routine of both client and patient. Special care should be given to prioritize these routines when arriving at a new narrative, likely involving a discussion to create a workable solution. A common example is an animal that does not take medication well. A pet who dislikes being pilled may begin to head in the other direction when she sees her owner approaching. It is well worth taking the time to problem-solve and find a way for the animal to receive medication while minimizing disruption to the human–animal bond. This can also increase compliance.

Reassuring the Anxious Client

Anxiety among clients is discussed in many places in this text, but it is so common, especially during the pandemic and its aftermath, that I believe it needs its own section. Anxious clients may be experiencing "anticipatory grief," which is discussed in Chapter Nine, or they may be focusing general feelings from their own life onto the health of their pet. Anxiety is not seen only among clients with seriously ill pets, it is seen in pet owners whose pets have only minor issues. Even people who don't normally engage in "catastrophic thinking" – or assuming the worst possible scenario will come to pass – can visualize dire outcomes befalling their pet even though the lump in question is merely a wart. Clients look to us for guidance, and one of the most helpful things we can provide is reassurance.

Here are some general guidelines for dealing with anxious clients.

- Remain calm. Try not to let any anxiety emanating from the client affect your own behavior. Hopefully, the client (and patient) will take their cues from you.
- Don't promise, but ease their minds. Although we can never "guarantee" a positive outcome, there are many ways to communicate that a client's concern is unlikely to be serious, such as:

  o I'd be really surprised if that happened.
  o I've never heard of that happening.
  o I'm not concerned about it.
  o Let's just keep an eye on it.
  o That would be really unusual/highly unlikely.

- Turn frustration into compassion. While you may resent taking the time to reassure a client who doesn't really have anything to worry about, consider how difficult it would be to experience their level of anxiety.
- Help the client to be mindful. If a person wants to dwell on hypothetical future scenarios that are not currently relevant, emphasize caring for the animal's present condition. Let them know there could be different options if the condition changes or progresses, which would be addressed at that time.
  - We'll deal with that down the road if we need to.
  - We don't have to worry about that right now.
  - There are things we can do if that does happen.
  - Right now, let's focus on dealing with this issue.

- Focus on positive signs. Let the client know that you think they are taking good care of their pet by highlighting indicators of good health other than their concerns.
  - You've done a great job getting him to lose a few pounds!
  - I'm glad the ear problem cleared up. All that cleaning paid off!
  - Her coat is so soft.
  - His heart sounds nice and strong! (Clients *love* to hear this.)

Realize that you can make a difference. Your words can have great impact on an anxious client's well-being, which can also positively affect their pet.

Common Sense and Nonsense

Some of veterinary practice consists of simply applying common sense. A client, stuck in their situation, may not realize a solution that seems obvious to you, an educated, objective observer. Sometimes our job is to condense the issue to the problem that requires a solution. It may appear to us to be something the client could have figured out on their own, but it can be hard to be objective about your own situation. An example would be feeding two animals separately by placing one in the bathroom (even a studio apartment should have a bathroom). Clients often insist they couldn't possibly feed two animals separately, yet once it is suggested many realize they could utilize their bathroom as a place for separation.

On the opposite end of the spectrum is the client who adheres to an irrational narrative that does not make sense. Dr. Launer suggests treating this as a "parallel narrative," the result of a different version of reality, and working to see where the two narratives could overlap or intersect rather than trying to convince the client to switch to your narrative, which is less likely to be successful (Launer 2018, p. 70).

Self-disclosure: Sharing Our Stories with Clients

How much do we reveal to clients about our own stories and experiences? Do we tell them our own beloved pet had the same disease as theirs? Share with them the type of food our own animals eat? Or discuss how we handled our own euthanasia decisions?

The sharing of our own stories is called self-disclosure, and it is beginning to be studied in human medicine. Currently, self-disclosure among physicians is controversial: some feel the patient–physician boundary should not be breached, while others feel self-disclosure can help humanize the practitioner and increase compliance and understanding in the patient (Arroll and Allen 2015).

Veterinary medicine differs from human medicine in that our position relative to our patient is more removed. Veterinary self-disclosure involves revealing our experiences in the role of animal caretaker, a role we share with our clients. This could make self-disclosure more valuable for veterinarians than physicians, as while an individual might not want to know the details of their physician's own colonoscopy, they may appreciate learning how their veterinarian's pet fared if they are considering the same procedure for their own animal.

After all, we aren't just veterinarians, we are also pet owners.

In this way, we are most like pediatricians who are also parents. One study has examined self-disclosure among pediatricians who discussed vaccinating their own children to vaccine-hesitant parents (VHPs). The study separated disclosures into personal self-disclosure (PSD), such as *I felt really comfortable vaccinating my own kids*, versus clinical experience self-disclosure (CSD) such as *We have lots of families who vaccinate here* (Lepere et al. 2019). Another type of CSD is a discussion of negative consequences, such as sharing the diagnosis or treatment of a patient who contracted the disease. This type of CSD should be familiar to veterinarians; examples are using a story about treating a parvo puppy to emphasize the importance of the parvo vaccine, or the physical example of a vintage glass jar above the cabinet containing a heart with heartworms.

Self-disclosure can also be done by support staff. When veterinary student Kate O'Hara worked at an animal hospital before veterinary school, she found a benefit to telling clients what heartworm preventative she used or the type of food she fed her own pets. "Some people just immediately relaxed when I did that...if you feel comfortable doing something with your own pet, it makes them feel more comfortable doing it with theirs."

Personal self-disclosure can change the dynamic to be less formal because you are talking to the client as a fellow pet parent and not only a doctor. Instead of being at the veterinary clinic, clients may feel as though they are talking to another dog owner at the dog park, or to someone on a social media chat group.

This should not serve to diminish the practitioner's status as a professional, but to humanize it. Clients may thus feel a more personal connection to their pet's doctor and may be more likely to follow their recommendations.

Self-disclosure as a Tool

Self-disclosure offers a chance of a more collaborative response than the top-down, "Here is what I think you should do" or "Here is what you need to do." Self-disclosure can vary from being superficial (*this is how I give my pet medications*) to far more revealing (*it was hard for me to make the euthanasia decision for my own cat*). It would make sense for a practitioner to feel comfortable self-disclosing about superficial topics before attempting to share something more personal. Furthermore, self-disclosure should always be done for the client's benefit, not as a way for a practitioner to work through their own feelings about a situation or decision. A vulnerable feeling after sharing a personal story can alert a practitioner that they may need to address their own feelings before sharing about that topic again. Self-disclosure should not change the topic of conversation from the client's pet to the practitioner's pet. It's best to keep self-disclosure brief initially; if the client wants to hear more, they will let you know. Finally, self-disclosure should not come with strings attached, and there should be no bad feelings if a client declines to follow a recommendation on a topic about which you have self-disclosed. We can put our stories out there without being attached to their outcome.

One way to broach self-disclosure with a client is to think of a variation of the phrase, "This is what works for me" or "This is how..."

This is how I give my cat pills.
This is how I remember to give monthly heartworm preventative.
This is how I took care of my dog when he was recovering from surgery.
This is how I came to my decision.

Another way to utilize self-disclosure is through the clinical experience model mentioned above, by bringing up a similar case you've seen. Instead of, "This is what works for me," you can say to the client, "This is what worked for another patient/client with a similar problem." There is no need to disclose personal information although you could mention nonidentifying factors such as the breed of the animal, its age, or certain details of the medical condition.

We have many clients who bring their cats into the clinic for fluid therapy.
This medication/therapy has helped many of our arthritic patients.
This worked well for another patient I have with Cushing's disease.
This is how many people arrive at the euthanasia decision.

As individuals, practitioners naturally have varying comfort levels sharing their own stories. When done on a superficial level, it shouldn't reveal much about us or feel like an invasion of privacy. After all, there is a big difference between sharing "this is what I did" and revealing "this is how I felt." While self-disclosure should never be forced, it can be a helpful way to connect with a client and help your patient.

A particular form of self-disclosure involves letting a client know if you've had a pet with the same problem as theirs. A client with a newly diagnosed diabetic cat may derive comfort from the fact that her veterinarian also had a cat with diabetes and feel more empowered to give her pet injections after hearing it was hard for her doctor too at first, but improved once it became part of their daily routine.

Clients occasionally request a hypothetical self-disclosure by asking, "Doc, what would *you* do if she were *your* dog?" This question is especially asked when the client is faced with a difficult decision like euthanasia and is seeking reassurance. This is a tricky request for practitioners, and many veterinarians dread the question. It can be difficult to relate to the client's unique circumstances, especially given our own perspectives, training and access to relevant resources such as discounted lab-work or professional services, and our ability to perform treatments at home. We also do not have intimate knowledge of their individual animal and its personality and preferences; even if we know them well, we do not live with them. However, as we will discuss in Chapter Eight's section *The Value of Reassurance*, reassurance from veterinarians has been identified as the most important support practice of veterinarians around the topic of euthanasia (Matte et al. 2020a). For this reason, it makes sense for practitioners to maintain a level of comfort with the question. The simplest response might be to let the client know how you would act if you were in their situation *at that moment*, with their available resources. There is no need to disclose that you might have scheduled your own pet for an ultrasound when the problem first occurred 3 weeks (or 3 months) prior.

Offering an answer to the question when it has not been asked (i.e. informing the client, "*I would make the same decision if she were my dog*") may provide reassurance to a client struggling with decision-making who may not feel comfortable or think of asking. Even a client who appears satisfied with their decision might benefit from this type of reassuring self-disclosure if the practitioner feels comfortable offering it.

Self-disclosure among veterinarians and staff is clearly an area that could benefit from research. Meanwhile, we can be mindful of how we use this strategy and how it affects our clients. Self-disclosure has the potential to help increase our client's confidence in both ourselves and their own abilities. In the age of internet "research," self-disclosure could help address the distrust some people have for professionals, bringing us one step closer to our patients and clients.

Case Story: *What You Said Helped Him*

Cocoa was a geriatric and well-loved chocolate Labrador whom I acupunctured for many months. Cocoa had two homes, as she spent time with both the young adult male owner and his retired mother, Connie, at whose home I provided acupuncture treatments. When the family made the decision to euthanize, I agreed to come to the son's home for the procedure. Connie told me ahead of time she would not be present, and we discussed how upset they all were about losing Cocoa.

At the son's home, he asked if we could perform the procedure outside, at a small beach area by a nearby pond. The young man carried the large dog to the beach, a labor of love, and we spread out a blanket. Then, he told me he was conflicted about euthanizing Cocoa as she was still eating. I told him I had made the decision to euthanize my own 14-year-old dog when she was still eating, and although a lack of appetite was often a sign that euthanasia should be considered, its absence did not mean euthanasia was the wrong decision for Cocoa. I also pointed out that Labs are known for maintaining their appetite in any situation. Connie's son nodded in agreement; the information confirmed what he already knew, and Cocoa died peacefully on the beach where she had loved to play.

A week or so later, Connie called to thank me for the card I'd sent and for speaking with her son. She told me he had been conflicted about the decision but had drawn comfort from my words about my own euthanasia decision while my own dog was still eating.

"What you said helped him," Connie told me.

The client had accepted my personal narrative as a way to support his own narrative.

Many times, I've said similar things to clients without knowing whether my words helped, and I realize some people may benefit and others may not. As long as a story does not make a situation worse, appropriate self-disclosure can be a valuable tool.

(Note: sympathy card writing will be discussed in detail in Chapter Eight).

Delivering Bad News

The delivery of bad news has been studied more in human medicine than in veterinary medicine. An article in the journal *American Family Physician* defined "bad news" as "information that may alter a patient's view of his or her future" (Berkey et al. 2018). Although we are not giving our clients information about their own health, we can consider that we are delivering information about an animal they likely consider to be a family member. In the case of a horse, working dog, or show animal, the person may also have personal goals that necessitate their animal to be healthy and fully functional. If a person's view of their future includes their pet, and their pet's health is at risk, this would certainly fit the definition of altering the person's future.

The sharing of serious findings involves an enormous and possibly unexpected change in the client's narrative, and they may initially be unable to fully comprehend what you are saying. As every client has different communication and coping skills, adapting your conversation to the client in front of you rather than delivering a "canned" speech is vital. Try to gauge their feelings and respond to them – are they ready for more information and a referral or are they still trying to take it all in? – and give the client time to process.

In an article I wrote for *Bark* Magazine entitled *How to Cope with a Serious Diagnosis* (Fine 2018a), I discussed ten helpful tips for clients once they have received bad news. One of my colleagues has found it helpful to give clients a copy of the article after delivering bad news, recommending that they read it while she is working up or stabilizing their pet or seeing another appointment. Here are the ten tips, changed to reflect the practitioner's perspective on how to guide the conversation:

1. Determine the Level of Urgency – It is important to communicate whether decisions must be made immediately, or if there is time for the client to digest the information first.
2. Put it in Writing – Consider writing down your findings and recommendations or have the client or an assistant write them down.
3. Consider a Specialist – You can discuss the potential benefits and costs of a referral and recommend a certain person or practice.
4. Consider Holistic Care – As above, you can go over benefits and recommendations of holistic treatments such as acupuncture or chiropractic care.
5. Beware of "Miracle Cures" and Other Online Traps – Many clients order expensive supplements that are not from reputable companies and are unlikely to help their pet; ask the client to check with you before purchasing anything.
6. When Doing Research Online, Choose Sources of Information Wisely – Let clients know that a website which is trying to sell them something may not be a good source of information. Consider giving clients the veterinarypartner. com website or another website you trust.
7. Remember the Real World – Although we may wish we didn't have to consider finances, most people do. We can assist clients with creating a plan that takes their financial situation and resources into account.
8. Consider the Animal's Perspective – People may react with horror to the thought of something like an amputation or enucleation, yet the animal may be able to maintain an excellent quality of life. Explain to the client what things are like from their pet's perspective.

9. Create a Bucket List – Even if time is short, there may be time to feed the animal their favorite foods if they are able to eat, and to say goodbye to loved ones. More time could mean more enjoyable experiences.
10. Reassure the Client – Many people are overwhelmed by the thought of making serious decisions about their pet's health, especially decisions regarding euthanasia. Remind clients that they know their pet best and that you are there to help support them and guide them through the decision-making process. Let them know they are not alone.

As every client has different communication and coping skills, adapting your conversation to the client in front of you rather than delivering a "canned" speech is vital.

Suggestions for Reflection and Discussion

- Can you think of a Problem in Parenthesis you've seen? How did it affect the client's narrative?
- Consider a few appointments you've seen. Write down the narrative the client came in with, and then the narrative created together with the practitioner, whether yourself or someone else.
- Have you ever self-disclosed to a client? How did it feel?
- Has a practitioner ever self-disclosed to you? What did you think?
- Has a doctor given you or a family member bad news? What was the experience like, and could it have been improved?

CHAPTER SIX

Recording the Narrative

The patient's record is an important document for many reasons: it helps the doctor to remember the patient and their symptoms, diagnosis, and treatment; it helps facilitate overlapping care with other practitioners; and ultimately serves as a legal document. In addition, the patient record literally tells the *story* of the patient's visit, as well as the reason for the visit and the treatment plan. It is the narrative not only of the patient but also of the caretaker, as told by the doctor and/or technician.

Many things are changing in veterinary medicine, and records are more likely to be digital than paper. This can affect the record, and in this chapter, we examine how those changes can affect the narrative, as well as the significance of the document itself.

Key Points

- As records become computerized, we should consider what we are losing by not having paper records, and look for ways to adapt electronic records to our needs.
- Human medicine is also struggling to incorporate more "story" into their medical records.
- Remember to include what is termed the "social history" in human medicine in the record, as well as other information important to a continued narrative.
- Consider adding a "C" to your SOAP to represent "Client Concerns," changing the acronym to SCOAP.

DOI: 10.1201/9781003126133-8

Why Keep A Record?

Historically, veterinarians kept records to remind themselves of how and when they treated an individual patient. When many practices were single-doctor practices, and lawsuits and board complaints rare or nonexistent, veterinarians often found they didn't need to write much to jog their memories. Thirty years ago, medical charts were not always even on full sized pieces of paper. Records often consisted of large index cards or sturdy paper folded in half and inserted into a small folder. Entries sometimes consisted of a single line, perhaps shorter than the "reason for visit" written by the receptionist, such as *Routine spay* or *Itching, Depo 1 cc.*

Now, records may be forwarded to specialists or emergency facilities, scrutinized by colleagues, and even act as a defense in a lawsuit. Veterinarians and technicians are trained how to write in the record, and many use a specific format or template to ensure nothing is omitted. Doctors and staff realize they may not be present when the animal is next seen, so records need to be as clear as possible in terms of the doctor's findings, thought processes, and plans, as well as the caretaker's words.

Timing

It didn't take much time to scrawl a line or two on a chart. Now, a thorough history, findings, and plan must be recorded, which is far more time-consuming. If written during the appointment, the doctor may miss some of the conversation with the caretaker, or the interaction between the animal and owner; the writer also runs the risk of appearing rude. Many clinicians, aware of this and of the clients and patients filling the waiting room, allow charts to accumulate and write in them at the end of a shift. However, this practice may allow certain details to escape memory.

The same problem exists in human medicine. Many of us have had the experience of a health provider typing into a computer like a court stenographer instead of making eye contact with us. Records should not take precedence over, or be created at the cost of, the practitioner–client–patient interaction. One solution is to jot down key words or phrases that can be used to fill out the chart later. Another is to take a few minutes at the end of the appointment to fill out the record, even if it means keeping the next patient waiting. Yet another is to have an assistant type or write notes to be transcribed later.

Human Medicine

Appropriate record-keeping has been an issue in the human medical field, where it is also affected by insurance and billing requirements. A 2020 article entitled *Restoring the Story and Creating a Valuable Clinical Note* states, "structured data from the electronic record are poorly suited to communicating an understanding of the actual person and their background, experiences, resources, challenges, hopes, fears, and goals (Gantzer et al. 2020)." The American College of Physicians has established a Restoring the Story Task Force, and there are even corresponding hashtags, #RestoringtheStory and #ReclaimClinicalNotes.

Dr. Charon is also concerned about the state of clinical notes, and points out that a hospital chart may be "written by dozens of health professionals but structured to minimize the idiosyncratic voice of any one physician," (Charon 2006, 146). In this way, the storyteller – the clinician – seeks to be as anonymous as possible, obscuring their own voice. Dr. Charon maintains that this habit arose at a time when medicine valued detachment, and may not be the best model for the profession going forwards (Charon 2006, 142).

Dr. Ronald Epstein addressed chart notes in his book, *Attending: Medicine, Mindfulness, and Humanity.*

> In medicine, patients' accounts of their illnesses are rich with inconsistencies, while chart notes are filled with seemingly coherent stories that confirm a diagnostic impression...too often, we shape the facts to conform to our beliefs.
>
> (Ronald Epstein 2017, 58)

Electronic versus Hand-Written

Electronic records are gaining in popularity and offer many advantages. They can incorporate lab records, eliminate problems with illegibility, and are easy to email and print. However, what are we losing?

Consider the paper chart of a well-known patient. It has a weight to it, this medical history that can be held in your hands. It can be measured. The thickness of the folder gives a clue to the health and age of the patient, as well as the dedication of the caretaker. The pages can be flipped through easily, revealing familiar handwriting. Coworkers can often identify the writer at a glance, without the need to search for signatures or initials. A couple of sticky notes may be evident, indicating an alert or reminder. A tiny bloodspot on a page from a syringe placed onto the record after a blood draw. A drawing of a corneal ulcer on one page, and a diagram of a lump's position on another. An exclamation of good news written in large letters, perhaps even underlined: *mass benign*!! A history not only of medical procedures, but of a life. Written by the doctors and staff who cared for a patient, a narrative of an existence, as related by loved ones over a lifetime of care.

Electronic records are less tactile, further removed. A one-page printout does not do the record justice. The electronic record may not lend itself to narratives as easily as a paper one, making it even easier to reduce an interaction between patient, practitioner, and client into a series of stock, reductionist phrases. What can we record about *this* patient, *this* client, and the unique world they inhabit?

Writing our notes by hand may also allow us to remember and understand them better. A study that looked at students taking notes on laptops versus by hand found that people processed information more when writing by hand. This is because students tended to type a lecture verbatim. Unable to write fast enough to keep up with the speaker, longhand note-takers had to consider *what* to write – they had to interpret what was important and what it might mean, which translated to better comprehension (Mueller and Oppenheimer 2014). One way to hopefully obtain this benefit when using computer records would be to jot down important points on a piece of paper before transcribing them into the computer record.

Writing the Worldview

Lately, there has been an emphasis on expanding the written objective findings being noted on every patient. Findings once assumed to be normal unless noted differently, such as whether the patient is ambulatory, are now often noted in the chart. While this is not bad practice, it is time-consuming and risks sacrificing other relevant information, such as what is called in human medicine the "social history" and the "family history." Dr. Launer's model of human narrative medicine (NM) stresses the importance of the family in patient narratives and states that "enquiry into the family dimension of people's lives is an essential part of a narrative approach (Launer 2002, 65)." In veterinary medicine, questions about the patient's family could explore questions such as Who does the patient live with – one person or an extended family? Where do they live – a third floor apartment or on a small farm? What is their daily life like – are they alone for much of the day or do they go to work with the owner?

Dr. Annie Wayne, Assistant Professor at Cummings School of Veterinary Medicine at Tufts University, suggests keeping notes on the client's personal history as many physicians do. The names of family members, their occupations, whether they live with extended family or have a child away at college, the presence of other pets in the home – all can be important information for the practitioner to be aware of, in terms of both caring for the patient and building and maintaining a relationship with the client.

As discussed in previous chapters, we need to view our patient in context, and our findings should be shared in the medical record. However, it is not enough to gather information in the medical record; it should also be interpreted (Murphy et al. 2016). If an animal has lost weight, for instance, has there been a chance in the pet's diet or activity level? Was the owner aware of the weight loss? If another dog moved in next door and the two dogs play together often, that can be noted in the record. If a cat is anxious because the clients moved recently, that should be in the record. If an obese dog spends workdays with the owner's parents who feed the animal continuously, that should be noted.

Electronic records lend themselves easily to templates, and there has been a recent trend toward the use of templates to record office visits. Yet, what are we losing when we stop the practitioner from writing a freeform narrative? For one thing, it is hard to realize what the visit was about. What did the client emphasize? What were their priorities? What did you spend most of your time discussing? How do you believe they felt at the end of the appointment? How did you feel? Were there Problems in Parentheses?

If a client declines a procedure or further testing and you know the reason, it should be included in the record. For instance, "Client declines dental cleaning at this time as she will be moving in a month and wants to wait until she is settled." Does the client decline something due to finances? If so, is it due to a lack of finances, or because they don't believe (or realize) the value of what you are recommending? For instance, a client may decline an echocardiogram because they think there would be nothing that could be done if their pet had a heart problem, not realizing many cardiac medications that are used in people are also used in animals. Or because they don't believe it's important? Or because now isn't a good time? Or because they've never brought a pet to a specialist and need to integrate that into their world view?

In your time with the patient and client, you may have learned important information about how to communicate with them, including the client's views and preferences. These should be stated in a nonjudgmental fashion, in such a way that the client would not be offended by reading them.

It is common for veterinarians to discuss multiple possible scenarios for ways to proceed with a certain patient. A cat who has vomited once may not require a full workup – unless the owner is leaving for a 2-week vacation the following day and wants to make sure her friend is okay before entrusting her care to someone else. All this should be documented in the record, not just the objective facts of the vomiting, physical exam findings, and any test results.

Client Concerns: Adding a "C" to form SCOAP

Veterinary student Elina Grunkina suggests adding a letter to the SOAP model of patient records to encourage the use of narrative. One way to include Problems in Parentheses and World View in the medical record would be to call them "Client Concerns" and list the concern along with an explanation. Adding a C for Concerns at the beginning of *SOAP* – forming *SCOAP* – would allow for a place to put those details that really describe who this person is, the nature of their relationship with their animal, and other factors relevant to their joint narrative which can inform diagnosis and treatment.

- Owner concerned about cost of procedure as her dog is already 10 years old and she's never had a dog live to be over ten before.
- Owner concerned about her ability to care for a diabetic cat; owner's mother was diabetic and had multiple complications.
- Owner concerned about her dog's vomiting especially because vomiting was her previous dog's first symptom of cancer.
- The cat lives with the owner's elderly mother and she's concerned about him scratching her because she takes blood thinners.

Record Identification

Veterinary student Daniel Markstein suggested a solution to the problem of all the records looking alike: different doctors could utilize different fonts and/or colors. Colleagues and staff members could then recognize at a glance which doctor the patient had seen, in the same way they recognized the handwriting on paper charts. Such a strategy would allow some individuality in patient chart writing while maintaining a professional and legible patient record.

Case Story: *The Chain Smoker*

At one house call appointment, I saw two cats with widely different personalities. The calm, overweight black-and-white tuxedo cat yawned as he was plucked from the sofa by his owner and carried to the kitchen table for me to examine. Afterward, he hung around for a chin scratch before calmly heading back to his still-warm spot.

The other cat, a small torti, had been confined to a bathroom before I arrived, as the owner knew she would bolt as soon as I came in the door. Thin and nervous, her pupils were dilated throughout the whole exam. "If she were a person," the owner stated, "She'd be a chain smoker." The description fit the little cat perfectly. In addition, it told me something about the owner: she had a keen sense of humor and was very observant about the personalities of her cats.

Case Story: *What's in a Name*

A house call client had three Beagles who were my patients for a couple of years. I hadn't seen them in quite some time when I received a phone call from an animal shelter. One of the dogs had been surrendered to the shelter, and a family was interested in adopting the dog. However, the potential adopters had small children and were deterred by the dog's name: Snappy. The shelter had been given one of my invoices with vaccine information, so they were calling to see if I had any insight into the name and whether I knew of a history of biting.

I laughed and told them not to worry. I remembered that the names of the family's other two dogs: Snippy and Snoopy (they were possibly named by children). Snappy had no history of biting or aggression that I was aware of.

Snippy, Snappy, Snoopy – these names represent the type of casual detail that may be penciled into paper record but not an electronic one – or that may not be written down at all, only remembered. In this case, my memory of Snappy's history helped find the dog a new home.

The Parallel Chart

In 1993, Dr. Charon invented something she terms the Parallel Chart as a place for students and practitioners to write reflective material they cannot include in the patient's official record. She asks her students to write at least one entry in a Parallel Chart each week, and stresses that it is not a diary, but part of clinical training; it is "narrative writing in the service of the care of a particular patient (Charon 2006, 157)."

Parallel charts are often used in NM medical student programs, where they are read aloud in small group settings (Charon 2006, 156). The use of Parallel Charts should be explored in veterinary medical schools, and their use is discussed further in Chapter Thirteen.

Suggestions for Reflection and Discussion

- What do you think are the pros and cons of electronic versus paper records?
- What do you feel is important to include in the patient record? What can be left out?
- Dr. Charon believes medical records may overly emphasize detachment and anonymity. Do you agree?
- The next time you write a SOAP, include a C for Client Concerns.
- Was there a time you wished more narrative information had been included in the chart?

Unique to Veterinary Medicine

SECTION THREE

Unique to Veterinary
Medicine

CHAPTER SEVEN

The Connection Triangle

It's a remarkable situation: a patient of a different species, unable to communicate in the language of caretaker or health professional. Yet the patient and client may understand each other quite well. How can we, as health professionals, best interact with them? And what is the nature of the relationship between the three of us?

In this chapter, we explore the unique and complex connections at the heart of the doctor (or staff member)/client/patient relationship.

Key Points

- There is a relationship between the practitioner and the human–animal bond as well as between practitioner and client, and practitioner and patient.
- It is important to try to preserve and support human–animal bond related routines, and this should be taken into consideration when making recommendations and cocreating solutions for patient care with clients.
- "Narrative glimpses" are snippets of stories, typically human–animal bond related, which can give valuable insight into the home lives of our patients.

The Connection Triangle: Three Distinct Relationships

Consider a triangle as a representation of the veterinarian–client–patient relationship. The practitioner is at the apex, with straight lines connecting to the other two individuals: the animal patient and the human client, as seen in Figure A.

DOI: 10.1201/9781003126133-10

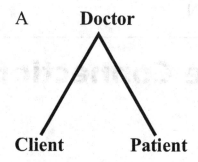

A   Doctor

Client   Patient

Now envision a line connecting the patient and client. This line represents their relationship, easily identified as the human–animal bond, a well-studied phenomenon (Figure B).

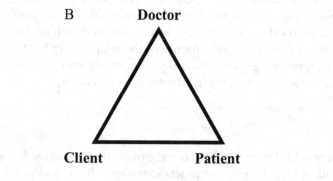

B   Doctor

Client   Patient

The relationship of veterinarian to the human–animal bond is represented by a line in Figure C.

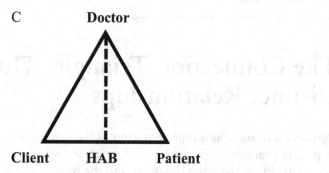

C   Doctor

Client   HAB   Patient

All three connections have the potential to affect us deeply, and we will explore the consequences of these relationships to ourselves in Chapter Eleven (Our Own Narratives). This chapter focuses on the nature of these relationships and how they affect patient care and client interaction.

The Human–Animal Bond

The human–animal bond has enormous significance in veterinary medicine. It is responsible for much of our income, unless we are in careers such as food animal, industry, or research. Along with other factors, it guides the choices of our clients. It is something most of us feel deeply on a personal level with our own animals. It is like a special language between human and animal. By understanding even a small portion of it, we can better communicate with the client and thus potentially improve our patient's health. The ability to witness the human–animal bond is more than a privilege, it is necessary for us to do our job. Yet, how can we have a relationship with a relationship?

The human–animal bond is something we feel a *connection* to. Each time we cry during – or after – a euthanasia, each time we smile at the happy reunion of a client picking up their hospitalized animal, each time we nod our heads as a person explains how their pet usually greets them at the door or eats with gusto but has failed to do so for the past 2 days, we connect with the human–animal bond. We cannot touch it as we can the points of the triangle, but a relationship is present, nonetheless.

The human–animal bond is always a unique and often a profound relationship; it will vary from person to person but also between two humans with the same animal, or one human with two pets. For some, the bond with their pet may be more important than many relationships with family members, especially family members they do not live with.

The bond may also vary depending upon how an individual views their animal – as a friend, partner, coworker, "fur-baby," or something not easy to define. Someone who hikes daily with their border collie may have a different relationship than a person who rescued a sick kitten to help fill an "empty nest." A bond may also change over time, and someone who wanted more of a "buddy" relationship with a dog when they were young may wish for a "family pet" type of connection when they have small children, and then may seek more of a close, emotional relationship with an animal after a divorce.

> The human–animal bond is something we feel a connection to. We cannot touch it as we can the points of the triangle, but a relationship is present, nonetheless.

What if the Human–Animal Bond Is Dysfunctional?

As practitioners, we treat pets from a wide spectrum of humanity. It is only natural that some of our clients will vary from being different from ourselves or what we consider "normal" to manifesting a form of mental illness. There may be times when we suspect or believe a client's bond with a pet is dysfunctional.

Our definition of dysfunction may reflect our own personal biases. Imagine a client who always arrives with her dog dressed in some type of outfit. If we are someone who delights in Halloween costumes and Christmas sweaters for our own pets, we may not think of it as strange, yet a coworker who would *never* consider putting clothes on her animals may think the client odd.

This is a good time to remember that our job is not to judge the client. If the animal is suffering or uncomfortable, of course the situation must be addressed. If the client's quirks are harmless to the pet, there is no need to interfere.

Even if we don't like the client, we can still empathize with their situation. They love their pet; we know how that feels. And if their animal is sick, we understand how painful that can be. Literature, film, and theater contain numerous examples of characters that we as readers and watchers don't necessarily like but still empathize with. We may appreciate certain aspects of their character but not others, which is how most people really are: some clients are terrific dog caretakers in every way except that they "don't believe" in heartworm preventative. Others may be chronically late for appointments, messing up the schedule, but always bring baked goods for the staff.

The Equine Patient: Pets with Purpose

Dr. Lauren Bookbinder, Clinical Assistant Professor of Large Animal Internal Medicine at Tufts Cummings School of Veterinary Medicine, makes an important point about equine patients:

> Horses are often more than simply pets for their owners. Most horse owners have their horse to fulfill some riding or athletic function, and these pursuits can be recreational, competitive, lucrative, or some combination of all three. So, while owners certainly love their horses like a pet, tied to this relationship is the expectation that the horse also fulfills it purpose. When this expectation is realized or exceeded, the bond between horse and owner deepens. When it is not, the bond fractures.
>
> (Lauren Bookbinder 2021)

How Connections Are Affected

We have now identified the three distinct relationships that the veterinary professional forms: with the animal patient, the human client, and the entity of the human–animal bond. For each leg of the triangle, there is the possibility for the connection to be weak. In each of the examples below, one area of the triangle is difficult to connect with, leading to a weak relationship. In these cases, more emphasis may be placed on the remaining legs of the triangle.

1. **Our connection to the animal might be weak** – This could happen with a difficult to handle or aggressive animal so that we dread an interaction with the pet. However, as trained professionals, it is not likely to affect our medical care as long as we are able to treat the animal safely.
2. **Our connection to the human–animal bond might be weak** – This often occurs when there is a weak bond between client and patient. For instance, if an owner brings in a sick animal who hasn't seen a vet in several years and the owner isn't interested in a workup. Of course, finances could be a concern, but it is usually easy to distinguish a financial issue from disinterest. If we know or suspect a weak human–animal bond we may feel badly for the animal, strengthening our connection to the patient.
3. **Our connection to the client might be weak** – Some clients are simply difficult to deal with, and may be entitled, arrogant, or even a bully. They may have an abrasive personality, constant complaints, or a history of ignoring our recommendations. Some people just "rub us the wrong way" and we can't figure out why. Alternatively, the client may be pleasant but could be "intense" or "needy"; so anxious about their pet that they repeat questions over and over, tying up doctors and staff members' time. In these cases, our connection to the human–animal bond is often enhanced. If we dread a client interaction, our consideration and respect for the client's bond with their animal, in addition to our concern for the patient, may help us relate and connect with them.

The following case story describes a situation where both the client connection and the human–animal bond connection were weak. While we are often faced with emotional situations regarding close human–animal bonds, the lack of a bond can elicit a different kind of sadness, and the doctor's compassion may act as a replacement for that of a bonded owner.

Case Story: *Nobody's Heart Horse,* by Dr. Lauren Bookbinder

Calliope was an upper-level dressage horse who was showing throughout the east coast as part of an elite show barn. Calliope had recently shipped into a 3-week long horse show and developed aspiration pneumonia during her travel. A few days into the show, she was lethargic, coughing and febrile. Pneumonia was confirmed and she was brought to a referral hospital.

Calliope and all of her medical decisions and communications were brokered through her trainer, Kris. The trainer had the owner's credit card information and was the point of contact for all decisions and communications. I knew the horses' owner by name, but nothing else.

At first, Kris "just wanted the mare to get better."

Great, I thought, *so do we!*

However, her tune slowly changed as I explained how long it can take for aspiration pneumonia to resolve, and how careful we have to be with these horses while their disease is active.

Just wanting the mare well morphed to: "well, she *is* for sale you know. We don't want to push her but she is supposed to get sold at one of these shows. I have buyers lined up to try her."

After only a few days in the hospital, the trainer had sent a trailer to pick the mare up and take her back to the show against medical advice. The mare was stable but still had active disease that could easily worsen if she was pushed. Thankfully, the mare was insured for a fair bit of money and I called her insurance agent to let them know about the "AMA" discharge. They called the owner and trainer, explaining that they would not pay for any of the medical care for the horse, or pay out for mortality related to pneumonia, if they did not follow medical advice.

The horse stayed in the hospital through resolution of her disease. I transferred off her case about halfway through her care. I was grazing her and brushing her during transfer rounds and told my colleague taking over her care about the communication challenges of this case.

"They want her back and showing as soon as we let them – she's nobody's heart horse."

I hope they sold her – maybe she is now.

Complicating Factors

Complicating factors can exist, typically for the client aspect of the triangle. There may be more than one owner, and different owners often have different approaches, ideas, and world views regarding the care of their animals. An animal may represent something for a person that may not have to do with the animal itself. This is often the case when a pet has previously belonged to a family member who is now deceased. In the story from Chapter Four, the dog with osteosarcoma represented the man's life before he married and had children. In the case of a horse, working dog, or show animal, the person's hopes and ideas for the future with that animal may play a large role in their decision-making and even how they view the animal in terms of its place in their life. If someone just lost a family member to cancer and the pet is diagnosed with cancer, the client will be understandably impacted by the pet's diagnosis.

Another complication could be the client's reaction to an emergent situation. As we touched on in Chapter Five, clients may become overwhelmed when they need to make unexpected life-or-death decisions for their pet. Sometimes, the client's whole personality might seem to change, as in the case story below.

Case Story: *Petunia and the Terrible Wonderful Client,* by Dr. Annie Wayne

I was still a new doctor, working at Angell in my first year of my ECC residency when I diagnosed Petunia, a 2-year-old Bulldog with a septic abdomen based on cytology of intra-abdominal fluid. She was very stable and bright, just had been slightly off to the owner. Ultrasound showed no obvious inciting cause for the infection, but she had been bred via artificial insemination by a breeder 2 weeks prior. When I explained to the owner that we recommended surgical explore to treat the infection and determine the source of infection, the owner reacted erratically. She was completely beside herself in disbelief that her relatively healthy-looking dog had a life-threatening disease, needed surgery, and that she would have to leave a deposit of several thousand dollars. I remember leaving the exam room thinking "this lady is nuts. I hope I never have to see her again." I was able to successfully convince her to send Petunia to surgery and she had a little hole in her uterus, presumably from the artificial insemination. She was spayed and recovered well. When the owner came to visit Petunia in the hospital the next day, I dreaded talking to her. But my interaction with her completely surprised me and gave me a new perspective on clients in the ER. She was wonderful! She was not crazy at all; she was a completely different person that I had met in the ER the day prior. We had a long conversation about Petunia and how grateful the owner was for the care she received. I stayed in touch with the owner long after Petunia recovered and when she came to the hospital for her preventative care, she always went out of her way to find me to say hi and bring me a card, picture, or treat. The experience helped me understand that when we meet owners in the ER, we meet them at their worst. Something has happened to their pet that is unexpected and interrupted their day. Often, we have to give them unexpected bad news and ask them to spend a large sum of again, unexpected, money. When owners react poorly or erratically, I remind myself of this owner and to give people some grace and space to process the information. I try to remember to not take it personally when owners react with anger to the information I give them and to partner with them to understand their situation, so I can help them make the best possible decision in a tough time.

Narrative Glimpses

Each human–animal dyad is unique, with a distinct language or flavor. We are offered the privilege of witnessing the closest of relationships, among the most intimate of many people's lives. It is often the small narrative glimpses related by owners which offer a window into their human–animal bond. Here are some examples:

- "She sleeps with her head in my hand."
- "Every Sunday, I make my special boiled dinner for us."
- "He loves cherry tomatoes, so we planted an extra tomato plant just for him."

Sometimes these stories are merely small, sweet anecdotes that brighten our days and strengthen our relationship with the human–animal bond of that patient and client. At other times, these glimpses may contain valuable information which could affect an animal's care, providing insight about the animal's condition or home life that you were previously unaware of. Consider the following example of a client named Lois who comes in with her dog Oreo because he is scratching.

Lois: Last night, Oreo and I were on the sofa having our ice cream after dinner like we always do and he wouldn't stop scratching. I mean, he's always been an itchy dog, but never this much....

What information can be gathered from the client's statement?

1. Oreo is more pruritic than he normally is.
   While it would be easy to stop there, there are other things to learn from what the client has said:
2. Oreo sits with his owner on the sofa after dinner.
3. Oreo and Lois eat ice cream together.

Item number 3 may elicit a "Wait...*what?*" moment; Lois may have just insisted that Oreo eats nothing except his special allergy-friendly diet. Concern may also stem from the fact that Oreo is diabetic, obese, and has gained weight since his last appointment. This information may illuminate a blind spot in the client's world, as she may not "count" ice cream as part of her dog's diet.

Further unbiased questioning would be needed to determine the full extent and nature of Oreo's ice-cream eating. We'll revisit Oreo and Lois in a little while, but first, we'll explore the importance of daily routines.

> Sometimes narrative glimpses are merely small, sweet anecdotes that brighten our days and strengthen our relationship with the human–animal bond of that patient and client. At other times, these glimpses may contain valuable information which could affect an animal's care.

Dr. Lynn Roy, practicing veterinarian and Student Wellness Advisor at the Cummings School of Veterinary Medicine at Tufts University, relates a wonderful story which illustrates the importance of the human-animal bond.

Case Story: *Human–Animal Bond: Stronger Than Ever,* by Dr. Lynn Roy

A few years ago, a tall, elderly gentleman entered the exam room with concern for his aging pet poodle, Joe. Joe was due for several vaccines and blood work which the owner wanted to complete before he started his "snowbird" migration to Florida for the winter. Discussing a history with the owner, he mentioned a reddened area near the anus which he had just noticed. On physical exam, I saw that this looked like a perianal adenoma or adenocarcinoma and confirmed on rectal exam that it extended deep into the anal sphincter. When I mentioned this finding to the owner, he became very quiet, then looked at me with tears in his eyes inquiring what we should do next. He then quickly added, "My wife recently passed away and Joe is all I have left of her." My heart went out to this man who was still mourning his late wife and I wanted more than ever to do all I could for Joe to extend his time with this compassionate owner. We then spoke about surgery and recovery and trying to fit it all in with his plans he already made for his "migration." While discussing our plans, the owner mentioned that he needed to be in Florida by a certain date as his son and daughter were going to meet him there to help him settle in. Hearing this, I paused to process that to this owner, Joe was all he had left of his late wife, but he was meeting his children (with his late wife) in Florida. I had to contain my smile and almost sudden outburst of laughter to realize that this dog gave his owner a closer bond with his wife than his own children. I certainly wouldn't want the kids to know this! But I am thankful for a dog like Joe (who did well with the surgery by the way) that provided love, comfort, and a strong human–animal bond that allowed his owner to grieve and live with an improved quality of life...even more than a human–human bond could apparently provide in this instance!

Daily Routines and the Human–Animal Bond

Why would the man in Dr. Roy's story not consider his children to be his main remembrance of his wife? It's likely because he hadn't lived with them for years, so they were not an intimate part of his recent daily routine with his wife.

Pets are a vital part of our daily lives, and this is reflected in the ways that our daily routines are woven around their presence and needs. These routines are important to preserve unless they are harmful to the animal.

Consider this passage from the 2016 novel *Lily and the Octopus* by Steven Rowley. The "Octopus" refers to a mass on Lily, the dachshund's head; a mass that her guardian, Ted, is so distraught about that he cannot even refer to it directly. The following passage occurs as Ted has come to terms with the fact that Lily's condition is terminal.

> There on the floor lies her empty bed. There in the bed is her paw-print blanket. There in front of the sink is the morning sunny patch she likes to lie in. There is the rack where we keep the pots and pans, the one that would swallow red ball, the one I'd find her stuck beneath trying her best to retrieve it, just haunches and a wagging tail. There is the vinyl breakfast booth; an understudy for her bed that was occasionally drafted for afternoon naps. There is the closet door that hides the garbage can, the door she would bat with her paw when she thought I'd been hasty in throwing decent food away. There is the drawer that houses her toys, the one she would give expectant looks to when she wanted to play. There was the pen that confined her for twelve weeks as she slowly recovered from surgery. There is the metal tin that holds her puppy chow and there on the floor is her bowl that twice a day gets filled. There is the back door she would guard with the menacing bark of a German shepherd whenever anyone came near. There is the mixer I used to make the batter that became her home-baked birthday cookies. There is the stove she would hit with a clang after her eyesight was gone. There is the corner she would stand and bark into once dementia had set in.
>
> (Rowley 2016, 257–258)

Ted's home is filled with memories of Lily, many involving daily routines – the twice daily filling of the food bowl, the morning sunny patch to lie in, the chasing of red ball. Routines such as these represent some of the building blocks of the human–animal bond.

The following case story is an obituary written by my client about her cat, Peanut. Pet obituary writing will be explored further in the next chapter, Guilt, Grief, and Shame.

Case Story: *Dear Pea kitty,*
by Mary E. Duane

From the moment I first laid eyes on you, I was smitten with love for you. You were so very tiny laying on the pillow in the spare bedroom – it swallowed you up. Instantly, you told me your name, Peanut. You were such a tiny package of life cat energy. I viewed you as a living cat angel.

Where did you come from that led you on that cold January day to let Val pick you up? You never released that secret, but I was so honored to have you let me be your human caretaker – partner. You never liked to be held, but you certainly let me hold you in my heart.

You certainly were an independent lady. When we moved together – you instantly made it a home for us. I could not imagine moving without you at my side. A house is a house unless you have a cat to make it a home. You filled those paws so very well. I remember you going around and checking it out – yeah – you sprayed the premises to bring us good luck. I look back now and figure you were assessing the mouse load. I only wish that I had kept track of all the mice you caught. Each and every mouse brought to me as a gift – thank you. How did you know that I am scared of mice?

I loved the way you stretched yourself full length on my legs as I watched TV at night. I loved the way you did a full "Vanna White" stretch each morning. I loved the way you snuck under the covers each night if even only for 10 minutes. I loved the way you were so passionate about licking the empty can of cat food completely clean. You were so darn cute.

I loved coming home because I knew that you would greet me with a quick pitter padder step and tiny peep. Quite often, I could see you in the front window looking out at me as I arrived home. Other times, as I opened the door, I would hear the plop from the bed and a quick padder on the floor to the kitchen to greet me. You rubbed against the table and looked happy to see me. You always brought a smile to my face.

When I was out in the yard tending bees or walking Buckie, I would look back and see you watching us in the window. You did such a great job of caring for us. I always felt that you were looking out for us.

Your facial expressions and tail inflections were clear statement of your opinion. You lived life on your terms and I respect that greatly. I will miss our full cat rub sessions on the bed post and bookcase when you needed it. You were such a passionate cat. Thank you for all that you taught me about living in the moment.

I feel such a loss on not hearing your purr or being able to pat you, but I am forever grateful that you allowed me into your heart. I know that we had something special. Your absence has left such a large void and your unique cat quirks will always be a reminder of our time together – Thank you my Sweet Pea.

Supporting Daily Routines

The above case story and novel excerpt demonstrate the importance of daily routines in our patient's and client's lives. With that in mind, let's revisit our patient Oreo.

Once it has been established that the dog does, indeed, have his own bowl of vanilla ice cream on the sofa each night, it is likely you will make a recommendation to Oreo's owner. As tempting as it may be to simply recommend eliminating the ice cream, any plan is not likely to be effective unless Lois is fully committed. From her original statement, you know it is a part of their daily routine and thus may be intimately intertwined with their human–animal bond. Lois's nightly routine with Oreo may represent the highlight of her (and his) day. If she were to agree, under duress, to give Oreo nothing to eat while she ate ice cream, she may still end up giving him his treat while feeling guilty or deceptive about it. In that case, Oreo would be no better off, Lois would have new, negative emotions associated with her favorite ritual, and her relationship with her veterinarian could be adversely affected, as Lois may feel as though she failed to take proper care of her dog.

A narrative medicine approach would involve offering suggestions in addition to the ice-cream-elimination solution. You could then work with Lois to create a solution that would preserve their routine while optimizing Oreo's diet. Perhaps Oreo's ice cream could be substituted with plain yogurt, or a few carrot pieces frozen into a cube of low-salt chicken broth. Alternatively, Lois could smear a tiny amount of ice cream around the bowl for Oreo to lick. Together, you and Oreo's owner can reach a compromise that preserves the human–animal bond, Oreo's health, and Lois's comfort level with her veterinarian.

Narrative Glimpses and Illness

When an animal is ill, the narrative glimpses may change, reflecting the client's concern.

"I went to three stores to get the food he likes."

"We cancelled our trip because we didn't want to leave him."

"I cook her food every morning, but I tell my kids they have to get their own breakfasts."

"Angus can't go up the stairs anymore, so my husband Jim has been sleeping on the sofa to be near him, and now Jim's having back problems."

Sometimes, narrative glimpses contain clues to a "Problem in Parentheses" (explored in Chapters Four and Five, Problems in Parentheses represent underlying client concerns that are often emotional, such as anxiety, fear, and guilt). In the above example, a client is concerned about her husband's health because he is sleeping on the sofa to be near the dog. This would warrant further, focused questioning: are the family members in agreement about the dog's care and treatment? Is there a way to get Jim back into his own bed, through medication for Angus (for pain or dementia), or through a lifestyle change? Ideally, these would be asked in a narrative style, using questions such as: How does everyone in the family feel about Angus's care? How does Jim feel about sleeping on the sofa, and how is it affecting the household? As with many situations, there are no right or wrong answers, as long as Angus's needs are being met and he is not uncomfortable.

Not Everyone Is a "People Person"

Not all veterinarians and staff are extroverts who naturally enjoy interacting with other people. Some are introverts, and many animal lovers (including doctors, staff, and clients) feel as though they are more comfortable with animals than people. That's okay! While some of us are energized by social interactions, others feel drained. Everyone arrives at work with a different skill set. Perhaps you are the "cat whisperer" at your clinic, or have a passion for cytology, or bring in yummy baked goods. Communication may not come naturally to all of us, but it can improve with practice.

If communication is a struggle for you, here are some tips:

- Identify which coworkers are skilled communicators and try observing some of their interactions with clients. Pay attention to their language, and the questions they ask people. Notice how the questions affect people. Some questions help people relax; these may be the same questions that prompt them to tell a story.
- Partner with one of these coworkers for office visits. A doctor-tech team with a technician who enjoys human interactions can work well, as the technician can explain clinic policies and medication instructions. The technician can also alert the doctor to any information she may have overlooked in the interaction.
- If you don't consider yourself a "people person," it's likely that the practitioner to human–animal bond connection is going to be even more important in your client interactions.
- Consider reading the book *Quiet* by Susan Cain, which deeply explores the value of introversion.

Suggestions for Reflection and Discussion

- Think of connections you have had to the human–animal bond between your patients and clients.
- What are some of your favorite narrative glimpses you have heard from clients?
- Write about some routines you have with your own animals, especially those we do daily – getting up in the morning, getting ready for bed, preparing and eating meals.
- How would you feel if some of the daily routines you wrote about had to be disrupted?

CHAPTER EIGHT

Grief, Guilt, and Shame

Guilt and Grief: Two emotions which are often intertwined and can lead to much suffering, especially when they are not adequately recognized or addressed. Guilt can also become internalized and leads to shame. In this chapter, we look at the grief and guilt experienced by our clients and explore how narrative medicine (NM) can help alleviate guilt and shame and soothe grief. The effects of these emotions on practitioners are explored in Chapter Twelve, Our Own Stories Part I.

Key Points

- Grief resulting from pet loss can be profound.
- We are problem solvers, but we can't solve grief. However, we can guide clients towards comforting rituals such as obituary writing to create a narrative about their pet.
- The guilt and shame clients experience surrounding death and euthanasia may be linked to a dysfunctional or false narrative regarding their ability to care for their pet.
- Reassurance from veterinary practitioners is a vital form of support for grieving clients.

Anticipatory Grief

Grieving often begins long before an animal's death. Anticipatory grief is the name for the grief felt when you think about or look at a loved one and consider – even feel – their loss while they are still alive. While it is often experienced when an

DOI: 10.1201/9781003126133-11

animal is ill, it can also be felt when they are healthy. As veterinarians and staff, we likely know this feeling all too well, especially after seeing a young patient die or experience a serious illness. We come home and greet our own pets, grateful to have them with us, painfully aware of the fragility of their lives.

Sometimes clients will feel anticipatory grief over a healthy animal, especially if they are old, or if they have experienced another loss in their life.

Not long ago, I was in the exam room with a client and her 7-year-old dog, Duncan. Dunc belonged to a breed which was very prone to cancer, and as a breeder herself, Duncan's owner was well aware of the propensity. Duncan stood on the exam table, practically glowing with health. His silky fur shone, his eyes were bright, his weight was perfect, and I knew his owner, Kelly, was devoted to his care.

Suddenly, Kelly began to cry.

"Two of his littermates have died in the past year…of cancer," she informed me.

"Oh Kelly, I'm sorry to hear that," I said, frowning in sympathy. I handed her a box of tissues.

"I'm just so afraid I'm going to lose him."

I couldn't tell her it wasn't going to happen. All I could do was to let her know that, at that moment, from what I could tell, he was in perfect health. Perhaps most importantly, knowing her distress was real, I could offer her my understanding, compassion, and support.

No decisions needed to be made about Duncan's care that day, although that is not always the case when we recognize anticipatory grief. Even as we make a treatment plan with the client, whether it's a referral to a specialist, scheduling a surgery, or dispensing medication, anticipatory grief is often in the room with us. While it cannot be made to disappear, it is better if it is recognized. Acknowledge the pain your client is feeling, then remind them of the good things: the treatments you will try, the time they have left, the continuing interest in favorite activities and foods. This may also be a good time to refer a client to a Veterinary Social Worker (see Chapter Eleven).

Case Story: *Pet Photos Helped Ease Our Anticipatory Grief* by Alice Oven

My husband and I adopted our King Charles Cavalier, JD, when he was two and he's now coming up to 10 years old. Although I grew up with dogs, my husband didn't, and JD is the first pet we've 'owned' as adults. He's a huge part of our life together and we care for him as we would a child; so much so that the thought of losing him is already painful, even though he's in glowing health. Once we were in a busy café talking with a friend (who's a veterinarian) about a dog she'd just had to euthanise, and my husband broke down crying just thinking about this happening to JD! This acute awareness that our time with JD is limited means that we try to appreciate every moment with him as much as we possibly can. One thing that really helped us is capturing the little intimacies and peculiarities of our relationship with him in a special pet photoshoot. Emily from *Pet Stories* came to our home in London and spent the morning with the three of us, taking beautiful photos that we'll treasure forever. It's a comfort to know that as JD gets older and less active, and even when he's gone completely, we'll always have that moment in time preserved, to look back on with a smile.

Should Clients Be Present for Euthanasia?

It seems like an age-old question, whether a conflicted client "should" be present for their pet's euthanasia. There's even a poem about euthanasia called *The Last Battle* (author unknown), which urges the client to "stay...till the end." Many clients have a strong desire to be with their pet, while others are clear in their preference to not be present. Occasionally, a client will be conflicted and want to discuss their options. These clients typically fall into one of two groups.

1. The client who would prefer to stay but is apprehensive about the process.
2. The client who would prefer not to stay but feels guilty about not being present.

It is important not to judge clients for their concerns and preferences. Losing an animal is difficult enough without feeling pressure to be present. We don't know the client's backstory regarding their comfort level with death and dying. Perhaps they were present for a family member's death and don't want to relive that, or they can't imagine being there at the time of death. An anxious client could also cause the animal anxiety and stress in their final moments.

For the client who is apprehensive, a review of what the procedure entails can help reassure the client that the process is typically a smooth one. It can be helpful to walk the person through each step of the process, so they know what to expect. With adequate support, these clients are typically happy to stay.

For the client who feels guilty about leaving, it can be helpful to offer permission for them to leave. "It's okay if you don't feel comfortable staying with Fluffy. I will be with him. Many people don't feel comfortable being in the room." You can give them options such as visiting with the animal after the procedure. If the client does stay at the clinic during the procedure, whether to visit afterwards or return home with the body, I make sure to seek them out after the procedure to let them know their pet died peacefully. If the client returns home before the procedure, I am sure to mention their good care of their pet in my sympathy card to help alleviate any guilt.

If the client seems conflicted and you aren't sure whether they'd prefer to stay or leave, offer "permission" for them to leave. If they want to stay but are hesitant, they will let you know.

The following 55-word story (a narrative form explored in Chapter 13) was written by veterinary student Michaela Roth for our narrative medicine selective at Tufts.

Case Story: *Twins*, by Michaela Roth

A little girl and her very best friend.
Her twin she'd always say.
Old, frail, grey hairs around the nose.
Time had come.
Too scared to say goodbye.
Couldn't say goodbye.

Years pass,
A woman cradling someone's best friend.
Reminds her of her twin.
It's okay if you can't say goodbye.
I can say goodbye.

The Story Behind the 55-Word Story

This is about the topic of euthanasia and how some people don't feel comfortable being present during it. When I was little, I had a golden retriever named Oliver. He was there from as young as I can remember. I use to always call him my twin because I am the only one who has red hair in my family and his hair was the same color as mine. When it came to putting him down, I simply couldn't bring myself to be there. Fast forward to my first time experiencing a euthanasia, a client had brought in this orange cat, and she had decided it was time to put him down. His name was Oliver. She was very upset because she couldn't bring herself to be there. So, I took the cat from her and walked him in the back, and I was the one who held him while he passed, and it was just a moment of realizing that I was now ready and able to do that for someone the way someone did that for me when I was little.

After a Loss

After the animal has died, there are many ways to grieve for them, and grief over the loss of a pet is becoming more accepted. Encourage clients to speak to friends, family, and coworkers who are likely to be understanding of the deep emotional pain of losing a dear animal friend.

For some people, the pain of losing an animal may be severe but not over-whelming; for others, the loss may be profound. The relationship with their pet may have been one of the most stable and important relationships in their life.

The grief of our clients may also be hard for us to handle because it is not a problem we can solve. While we can offer support, understanding, and resources, grief is not a problem we can fix.

Unfortunately, the relationships people have with their animals are sometimes trivialized or even mocked by family, friends, or coworkers.

"It's not like she was a person,"

"It's just a cat."

"Are you *still* upset about that?"

The relationship may have been a primary one in the person's life, yet they may not have even been able to take a day off from work to grieve. This is called Disenfranchised Grief, and is also discussed in the chapter on Veterinary Social Work.

A familiarity with available resources is especially helpful, as they can then be offered to clients. Even if a client chooses not to take advantage of any of them, just knowing they are available can help a person to feel less alone, as the very existence of the resources validates their grief; other people must also feel this way if those resources are available. Many veterinary schools have pet loss support hot-lines and lists of books, articles, and other resources for both children and adults. In addition, it can be helpful to become familiar with veterinary social workers or therapists in your area who specialize in pet loss and the human–animal bond.

> For some people, the pain of losing their animal may be severe but not overwhelming; for others, the loss may be profound. Their relationship with their pet may have been one of the most stable and important relationships in their life.

Grief Rituals to Recommend

Rituals can be an important part of grieving and may allow people to mourn in pro-portion to their sense of loss. Here are some ideas for rituals to suggest to clients:

- Set up a small shrine, including photos, any sympathy cards, and perhaps a candle.
- Say a prayer or a blessing in whatever religious or spiritual fashion you choose.
- Display or plant flowers in your pet's memory.
- Create a "memory book" photo album of your pet's life.
- Create a photo collage of your pet and frame it.
- Make a donation to an animal related charity or donate some of your pet's leftover food or former possessions.
- Hold a Celebration of Life and enjoy some food with family and friends as you share stories about your pet.
- Write an obituary, which we will explore in the following section.

Writing an Obituary

Obituary writing is a comforting ritual for people that we can also use for animals; it has been a helpful activity in my own life, and I have long recommended it to clients. In addition to being a traditional activity after a loss, it is also an opportunity for the client to tell and share their animal's story, which can be deeply healing. It is NM for the client: a way to provide a record and acknowledgment that this individual existed, they were real, and a part of them lives on in our memories. Obituary writing is also a positive activity a grieving person can focus on during what may be a difficult and lonely time.

The following Guide to Writing a Pet Obituary is also available on my website. The case story *Dear Pea kitty* in the previous chapter is an obituary written by one of my clients.

Guide to Writing a Pet Obituary

Our pets feel like family members, and we grieve them the same way. Your pet's obituary may never make it to the local newspaper, but it can still provide an enormous amount of solace for you and any other family members or friends.

There is no right or wrong way to write an obituary for your pet. The goal is to put something down on paper – or computer – to memorialize your beloved animal, and your relationship. No memory is too small or insignificant; it is the tiny, intimate details that many people miss most. You can do this individually or together with other family members or friends. You can do it a little at a time or all at once. You can make your obituary as high tech (all computerized) or as low tech (handwritten) as you choose, but I do recommend that you print out a copy if you write something on the computer, so you have something tangible and real rather than solely virtual.

There is also no right or wrong time to write about your pet. Even if they died many years ago, it may still be helpful to write an obituary for them.

Here are some ideas of what to write about to get you started.

- Write out a list of your pet's nicknames (possibly including how they came to be)
- How did you obtain your pet? Describe the first time you saw them.
- Who do they leave behind? Include family, any other animals, and friends.
- Did you know your pet as a puppy, kitten, or young animal? What was your pet like as a youngster, or when they first came to live with you?
- What were your pet's favorite games, toys, and activities?
- What was your pet's favorite food?
- What places did your pet travel to? What was their favorite place to visit?
- Where was your pet's favorite place to sleep?
- What was your pet's favorite time of year?
- What was your favorite part of your daily routine with your pet?
- Describe your pet's personality, including good and bad qualities (i.e., sneaking food off the counters). What mischief did your pet get into?
- What were your favorite personality traits and quirks?

Once you have created something, here are some ideas for what to do with your pet obituary.

You can email your writing to friends and family or post it online on social media to let people know about your loss. You may then wish to invite people to share their own memories of your pet. You can also send a copy to your veterinarian, groomer, pet store owner, doggie daycare provider, dog walker, or anyone else who has been a part of your pet's life. If you choose to make a donation in your pet's memory, you may choose to include a copy of your pet's obituary.

You can print out or create a copy of your obituary and put it somewhere in your home along with a picture of your pet, a candle, a favorite toy, and any other mementos to create a small shrine. If you choose, you can purchase special, decorative printer paper to print your words onto. You can frame a copy, or place one in a drawer, or with your pet's ashes, if you have chosen to keep them. You can keep a copy with you, in your pocket or in your wallet or purse.

If you have children, you can give them each their own copy, and they can decide where they would like to keep it. They may choose to personalize their copy with drawings or additional words.

However you choose to share and keep your pet's obituary, you will have created a special document to help preserve your precious memories of your beloved pet (Fine 2018a).

Sending a Sympathy Card

Sending a sympathy card is an important practice and should not be skipped. In some cases, it may be the only expression of sympathy a client receives. In addition, our words can do much to help assuage any guilt a client may feel (more on that soon).

We say or write the words a person may cling to in their bleakest moments: *You did all you could. You made the best decision.* Or simply, *it was time.*

Sympathy card writing can be cathartic for us, but also difficult, especially as it never seems to stop; our patients continue to die. Spend some time picking out cards with phrases that resonate with you, so if there's a day when you want to say something profound and personal but the words won't appear, you can simply sign your name. Some people find it helpful to keep a list of phrases that are meaningful to them and that they have used in the past. Examples of such phrases might be,

> *I am so very sorry for your loss.*
> *Fluffy was such a great dog.*
> *I know you must miss her very much.*
> *You took such good care of Fluffy.*
> *Fluffy was blessed with a loving family.*
> *I know it was hard to say goodbye to Fluffy.*
> *It is never easy to say goodbye.*
> *You made the best decisions for Fluffy.*
> *Please know that we are thinking of you.*

The Lingering Loss

Grief isn't linear, and many people mourn the loss of an animal for years. The deceased pet remains a part of their life, and sometimes, they want to talk about them. Just being back at the clinic or seeing you or other staff members may trigger certain memories. And, some people may not have anyone else they can talk to about their animal, or anyone in their life who understands the depth of their grief. Listening to a client reminisce about a deceased pet may not seem like part of our job description, but we are in a unique position to provide solace where it is greatly needed. And, we can listen to these narratives without the need to problem-solve; just listening with attention and compassion can be enough.

Case Story: *I Still Miss My Old Cat*

During the pandemic, appointments at my workplace were checked in "curbside" and clients were not allowed in the building. However, the clinic was fortunate enough to have two exam rooms with windows directly facing the parking lot, and Dr. Mulcahy, our clinic's chief of staff, set up a roped-off area six feet from the windows, under an awning with some chairs and even some potted plants. We were then able to speak to our masked clients "face-to-face" through the window instead of over the phone.

Once we were back to seeing wellness appointments, I saw a young cat for a routine checkup. The elderly client stood by the window and I tried to speak loudly through my mask as she seemed a bit hard of hearing. Every so often, a truck rumbled by on the road, causing us to pause in our conversation until the noise had passed.

The cat's exam was unremarkable, and I spoke to the client as my technician brought the carrier back outside and handled the payment.

Suddenly, the woman changed the subject.

"I still miss my old cat," she told me.

"Oh, of course you do," I responded. I'd been about to get up from the stool I'd placed by the window, but I settled in. I could tell she needed to talk, and I wanted to hear the story of her "old cat." I leaned forward on the windowsill as much as I could to let her know I was listening.

"She was such a comfort to me when my husband was dying. He died of cancer a few years ago. And that cat knew, she knew he was sick, and she was such a comfort to him and to me."

I told her that I was sorry for both of her losses.

"Now they're both gone. I'm so glad I have this one, but I still miss the other one."

I said that I understood and tried to validate her grief as best I could. We spoke for a few more minutes, and she thanked me for listening. I couldn't touch or hug this woman, or even stand close to her, but I hope that by receiving her story through the window I helped honor her memory of her beloved cat.

Guilt versus Shame

Guilt and shame are often used interchangeably, but they do mean different things. As shame researcher Dr. Brené Brown writes,

> The most important difference to remember between shame and guilt is that the thoughts that accompany shame are focused on the self ("I am bad"), whereas thoughts associated with guilt focus on a specific behavior ("I did

something bad") … Although people tend to assume that shame and guilt are both "bad," research has revealed important differences between the two. More specifically, shame tends to have negative outcomes whereas guilt can be adaptive and helpful.

Brown (2019).

While guilt can prompt a person to make amends or take steps to prevent a situation from recurring, shame can become internalized and develop into a lonely, private, and often long-lasting burden.

Guilt, Shame, & the Negative Narrative

Guilt is an emotion that often arises when someone dies, especially an animal the person is responsible for. However, it can also be a feeling that is experienced throughout the life of the animal. In both cases, it is often undeserved.

One day at the clinic, I saw a little dog for wellness checkup.

"While he's here," asked the owner, "would you mind looking at his back leg? He limps sometimes, after he's run around a lot." She pointed to his right hind leg and winced. "I think it's because I stepped on him when he was a puppy," she added softly. That was the narrative she believed; I could see it in her eyes.

I examined the dog's leg.

"He has a kneecap that moves in and out, which is common in little dogs," I told her. "He was born with it, but the occasional lameness can show up when he's a bit older like this. He may have some arthritis there. It has *nothing to do with* you stepping on him." I recommended he lose a pound or so and we discussed his diet. I felt badly that she held herself responsible for her dog's occasional lameness. Even though she'd stepped on him as a puppy, it had surely been accidental. How much pain had she inflicted on herself by repeating this narrative to herself every time she saw him limp?

It's unlikely that my comments were able to cure the woman's guilt. Perhaps her tendency to feel guilty stretched back to childhood, to a world in which she was regularly blamed for things that were not her fault. Perhaps she regarded anything that happened to her dog as being her fault. However, it is possible I was able to alleviate some of her guilt and shame if only for a short time.

Consider these excerpts from the 2018 novel *The Friend* by Sigrid Nunez. In the book, the unnamed narrator adopts the dog of her late friend and former lover as she mourns his loss.

When people ask me why I stopped having cats I don't always give the true answer, which has to do with how the ones I did have died. Suffered and died.

The narrator causally relates her decision to stop having pets to her experiences around the deaths of her previous cats. She continues:

> The intolerable thought that your dog, who believe you are God, believes you have the power to stop the pain, but for some reason (did he somehow displease you?) refuse to do so.
> The trip to the vet, the diagnosis, well, that at least, at last. Surgery, drugs. (Stop spitting out those goddamn pills!) Hope. Then doubts. How do I know if she's in pain, and how much pain? Am I being selfish? Would she rather be dead?

The narrator places an enormous amount of pressure on herself: can she live up to the absolute faith she believes her animal places in her? The answer, almost by definition, appears to be "no." Many people feel incredible pressure around the decision to euthanize and feel ill equipped to make that decision.

The narrator then describes the euthanasia procedure of her 19-year-old cat, who was ill and suffering. When the veterinarian has trouble with the injection, her cat looks directly at her.

> I'm not saying this is what she said, I'm saying this is what I heard:
> Wait, you're making a mistake. I didn't say I wanted you to kill me. I said I wanted you to make me feel better.
>
> (Nunez 2018)

The narrator clearly believed she had failed her cat despite providing her with a good home for 19 years and following her veterinarian's recommendation for compassionate euthanasia. The feeling of failure has a long-lasting effect on the narrator as she does not get another cat.

The narrator also describes another cat she lived with for 20 years, "longer than I've lived with any person," illustrating how important and primary her relationships with her animals were to her life. How many of our clients put similar pressure on themselves, especially around the issues of euthanasia and death?

When people believe they failed a previous animal, their memories of their beloved pet may become intermingled with regret and shame. This shame is woven into the narratives of their lives with the late animal, and often affects the narrative of current pet(s) as well, as they don't want to repeat what they felt were their own past mistakes. "I waited too long with my last one…I don't want to make that mistake again," is a common refrain from clients who feel this way. It may help for us, as practitioners, to recognize that a client's self-narrative – which is related to their world view – may be dysfunctional. For instance, how does that person understand disease causation? Some people may feel their pet's diagnosis is somehow related to something bad they themselves have done. It is also common for people to ask themselves what they could have done to prevent their pet from becoming ill and fault themselves for not realizing sooner that their pet was sick. While many people move on from such questions, some do not.

The Value of Reassurance

Pet loss can be incredibly painful, and many people talk about how they "can't go through this again" which is why they "just can't get another pet." How many people who say this are affected by dysfunctional narratives? As evidenced in the above story, narratives around euthanasia can last for years, even a lifetime. As practitioners, we can watch for dysfunctional narratives and try to reassure pet owners that, in most cases, their action or inaction did not contribute to their animal's illness. Although we may not be able to change a client's dysfunctional narrative, we can address them. For instance, a person may receive enormous comfort from something like the following words:

> I remember when Rosa was sick; you took really good care of her. It's easy to look back and think that you could have made different decisions. But you really took her needs into account. You made the best decisions you could with the information you had at the time.

Reassurance regarding euthanasia can be immensely important to clients. One study found that "Pet owners, concerned about their choice to euthanize, often phoned veterinarians to seek reassurance that they had made an "appropriate" and "reasonable" decision (Morris 2012)." Another study involved an online questionnaire which was informed by an initial round of focus groups with pet owners. The questionnaire was administered to over 2,000 participants worldwide (the majority residing in North America) who had experienced the euthanasia of a companion animal over the past 10 years. As part of the study, participants were asked to rank 10 forms of support practices used by their veterinarian at the time of euthanasia. These forms of support were identified through a previous study of veterinary professionals' emotional support practices during end-of-life care (Matte et al. 2020b).

Ranked first was "Reassurance (e.g., You did the right thing)" (Matte 2020a). However, the study demonstrated that while a slim majority reported receiving reassurance, many did not. The authors concluded,

> Only 59 percent of pet owners felt they received reassurance from their veterinary professionals. These findings suggest that there may be opportunities for veterinary professionals to use reassurance more often when supporting pet owners. Examples of reassurance may include reassuring the pet owner that they have made the right decision, that the veterinarian will do their best to ensure the companion animal passes away peacefully and reassurance that

the veterinary staff are there to support them. Reassurance intends to promote a sense of confidence in the pet owner around their decision, the process of euthanasia and the commitment of their veterinary professionals. The use of reassurance may enhance participants' satisfaction with the emotional support they receive and in turn their overall satisfaction following companion animal euthanasia.

(Matte 2020b)

It is important to realize that there is much room for improvement in offering reassurance to clients surrounding euthanasia, especially as reassurance was identified as the most important form of emotional support. While a practitioner should never feel pressured to tell a client "You did the right thing" if they are not comfortable saying so, just the expression of that simple phrase can provide enormous comfort to an individual grappling with excessive or irrational guilt.

Another way to consider the importance of reassurance is to examine how conflicted clients attempt to reassure themselves about a decision to euthanize. It is not uncommon for clients to consult animal communicators, which veterinary student Caitriona McIntyre, who has worked with animal communicators in the past, explained can be a way for a client seeking spiritual guidance to "find comfort in making a difficult decision by obtaining their pet's permission." While I used to feel uncomfortable if a client sought out an animal communicator, I now realize how troubled the client likely is by having to make the decision, and I hope the consultation will bring the client some peace.

The Narrative Shift

Dr. Katherine Nickerson from Columbia used a term called the narrative shift which I find helpful. The client's narrative may be built on many previous experiences including their childhood, previous pet experiences, and previous experiences with both animal and human health care. While it's unlikely you will completely change their world view, you can aim for a "narrative shift." The effects of your words and actions may be incremental, but you can help, for instance, reassure an anxious person that they are doing the best for their pet or support a frustrated client by repeating that their pet should be feeling better soon.

Dr. Launer also believes that the result of a conversation might simply be a person thinking of things differently.

Often, the change that occurs in the conversation is simply a shift in thinking, rather than a concrete decision. For instance, someone may realise in the course of a conversation that what they were already thinking or doing was right all along, and feel more comfortable about it.

(Launer 2018, 41)

Dr. Wayne likes to think of this type of result as "planting a seed" regarding euthanasia or another difficult decision, or a matter to address at another time. In an urgent or emergent care setting, this may involve addressing the most urgent problem while recommending follow-up care later or with another provider.

Another way in which we can consider a "narrative shift" is our own spoken response when a client is faced with a difficult decision. Consider the situation of an ill geriatric patient for whom you are discussing with the owner whether to euthanize or perform a workup (or continue with treatment). In some situations, you may feel that a certain course of action would be preferable, but many times, either one would be appropriate, and it is really up to the owner to decide. In that case, you would likely present both options as equally acceptable. Once the owner has made a decision, however, especially a decision in favor of euthanasia, it may be possible to shift your spoken narrative to reinforce the client's decision. This would never involve saying anything you don't believe. But, for instance, if the animal is clearly uncomfortable, you could reassure the client by repeating that fact and telling them they are making the right decision for their pet, even if a decision to pursue treatment would be equally right in your opinion. If a client chooses to pursue a workup or referral, you could reinforce the reasons for obtaining a diagnosis. The reason for reinforcing the client's decision is to shift the narrative toward the client making a "good" decision as opposed to simply "a" decision; this can help prevent or minimize any guilt or shame the client may later experience for deciding to euthanize their pet rather than treat, or for pursuing a workup in case the animal does not recover.

Research also needs to be done to better understand people's dysfunctional narratives around their pets and how they might affect pet owners and their decisions about obtaining and treating future pets.

> The reason for reinforcing the client's decision is to shift the narrative toward the client making a "good" decision as opposed to simply "a" decision; this can help prevent or minimize any guilt or shame the client may later experience for deciding to euthanize their pet rather than treat, or for pursuing a workup in case the animal does not recover.

Case Story: *I Should Have Noticed It Sooner*

Lorraine lived alone in a cute little cottage with her cat, Blackie. Blackie was getting older, and we had diagnosed him with hyperthyroidism, but he had been doing well on his medication. Lately, however, he'd been drooling, and Lorraine had asked me to come over and take a look at him.

A friendly kitty, Blackie was in the kitchen when I arrived, and I put my things down and went over to him. As soon as I touched his chin, I could tell there was a mass on one side. I lifted his head and looked at him straight on, noting the asymmetry on the lower jaw. The mass felt bone-hard to the touch, and I knew it was not an abscess.

Reluctantly, I told Lorraine what I had found.

"I should have noticed it sooner. I'm a bad pet owner," she chastised herself.

"Lorraine," I told her, "Of course you aren't!

You are not a veterinarian with over twenty years of experience. The mass is hard to see, there below his chin. Besides, you see him every day, and that makes it really hard to notice changes like this. This is *not your fault*."

As with many clients, Lorraine's first impulse was to blame herself.

Fortunately, Lorraine spoke her fears out loud and allowed me to reason with her. I had treated her cat for several years and been in her home, which surely helped with her comfort level. As we talked, she acknowledged the truth in what I was saying. Not every client will be as forthcoming as Lorraine, yet many people's first response to a bad diagnosis is to blame themselves.

Suggestions for Reflection and Discussion

- Have you experienced anticipatory grief, as a practitioner or in your own life?
- How do you feel about writing sympathy cards: is it a chore or a way to explore your own emotions?
- Have you ever written an obituary for your own animal?
- Think about a time you talked to a client who felt guilty.
- Have you ever shifted your narrative to reinforce a client's decision?

CHAPTER NINE

Narrative Medicine and the Workplace

The people we see the most, even more than our clients and possibly our family members, are the people we work with – our work family. In this chapter, we examine how narrative medicine (NM) can enhance our connections with our coworkers, increasing cohesion and minimizing dysfunction. We will also examine how we can work together with the goal of excellent patient care and client communication. Finally, when a well-known patient dies, the loss can affect the entire staff. Employing some NM strategies in the workplace can help increase staff wellness and decrease burnout and compassion fatigue.

Key Points

- It is helpful to understand our coworker's narratives.
- Staff can make others aware of any connections to clients and patients to increase knowledge of client/patient narratives.
- Recognize that the entire team can grieve over the loss of a patient.
- Staff tasks can be uniquely stressful, so it's important to realize each other's job responsibilities and how demanding they can be; something other team members may not fully appreciate.

Be Aware of Each Other's Stresses

Each clinic member has a unique position within the dynamic of the workplace, and each position has its own demands and responsibilities, which can be difficult for other team members to understand, especially if they have never held that position. In addition, due to the nature of practice, each role has things which are not under the individual's control, which can create stress. For instance, an associate doctor

DOI: 10.1201/9781003126133-12

may wish for a more reasonably booked schedule, while a receptionist may wish for more flexible doctors. Part of narrative medicine is the ability to consider another's story, and this includes the stories of our coworkers. You may know your coworkers' job descriptions, but not know what it's like to spend time in their shoes. In this section, we explore some of the common responsibilities of team members in a small animal clinic. Perhaps if we understand their stories better, we can work toward being less judgmental and more accepting of our coworkers' decisions and actions.

Receptionists

Experts at multitasking, receptionists are the first line into the clinic; the first voice a client hears when they call or arrive at the clinic. They often handle in-person clients at the same time as people calling on the phone (and possibly texts and emails as well). Clients quickly become agitated when their pet is sick, so front desk staff interact with many people who are anxious, worried, upset, or even angry. Many of us are familiar with the phenomenon of a client acting rudely to a receptionist, then turning on the charm for the doctor. Some clients may insist on being seen, and whether an animal is really in need of being squeezed in or double booked can be impossible to tell until the animal is examined. Receptionists are frequently placed in a difficult position between an anxious client who wants their pet to be seen and an annoyed, overworked doctor, who is stressed about the possibly unnecessary addition to the schedule.

Veterinary Technician/Nurse

Veterinary technicians or nurses typically have multiple responsibilities to juggle during the course of a work day: running lab work, assisting in patient care, seeing tech appointments, interfacing with doctors, and speaking to clients. Much like doctors, they may have to triage their tasks during the day to determine which are more important at a given moment, helping the doctor with an emergency versus treating a sick hospitalized animal.

Office Manager

An office manager may manage multiple tasks including ordering supplies, arranging schedules, taking inventory, and dealing with difficult clients. In some clinics, the office manager is the point person to deal with disputes or complaints from staff members, putting an additional layer of stress onto the job.

Associate Doctor

An associate doctor works at the practice but is not the practice owner or manager. Associates are directly involved in seeing appointments, patient care, and performing surgeries. Some are on call. While they may appear to have more control than other positions at the clinic, they are likely not in control of their schedules, and they do not control how clients choose to treat their animals. They make recommendations that clients may decline to follow. While other staff members play vital roles in veterinary appointments, doctors are tasked with deciding what to recommend to clients, interpreting results, delivering unwelcome news, and facilitating euthanasia procedures.

Veterinary Assistant

A veterinary assistant may help a doctor during appointments or assisting with inpatient care. Veterinary assistants may witness traumatic events for which they may not have sufficient training or background to help them process. For instance, they may witness the arrival of a patient that has been hit by a car and bleeding badly and then have to "bag" the body after the animal has died or been euthanized. They may not be in control of their daily tasks at the clinic, which can be stressful.

Practice Owner/Chief of Staff

The practice owner or chief of staff is responsible for the entire clinic; if a patient dies or a case is mishandled, they have the ultimate responsibility even if they were not in the building at the time. Management and business tasks can take enormous amounts of time in addition to the clients this doctor typically sees. In order to get everything done, it may be necessary for this doctor to delegate responsibilities, which can cause friction among staff members.

Case Story: *The Client Who Wouldn't Euthanize*

Shasta was a toy poodle who was already geriatric with multiple problems when she became recumbent. Practice owner Dr. Mulcahy saw the dog weekly for acupuncture and had regular conversations with the client regarding the animal's quality of life. The client, however, was resistant to the idea of euthanasia and insisted her dog would pass "in her own time." Dr. Mulcahy was frustrated by the client's denial of the dog's condition and tried to prescribe medications to make the dog as comfortable as possible. The dog was eating and not in obvious pain but seemed mentally confused and appeared to be physically wasting away.

It was difficult for everyone at the clinic to see this dog; they all felt the dog should have been euthanized. When Shasta arrived weekly for acupuncture sessions, staff members often complained to the doctor that she should tell the client to euthanize her dog. Dr. Mulcahy felt badly that she was unable to convince the client and she was also hurt by the judgment of her staff. However, she knew that the acupuncture provided the dog some relief, so she kept scheduling the appointments.

Eventually, prompted by Dr. Mulcahy, Shasta's owner did make the decision to euthanize. Technician Cindy Moss was present during the procedure and was stunned when the dog's owner stated, "I hope I'm not going to hell for this." Cindy realized that the owner fully believed the decision went against her religion and she would be judged by God for euthanizing her suffering pet. Cindy then understood just how difficult it had been for the doctor to convince this client to euthanize her dog.

Personal Narratives

In addition to clinic worker's individual job stresses, everyone has a unique personal narrative. One person may have a chronic illness or care for someone at home who is ill. Someone else may be contemplating getting married or divorced. Everyone has their own triggers and perspectives. Recalling the background and context of someone's life can help someone feel compassion rather than frustration if a coworker is unusually tired (maybe they were up late with the baby last night), distracted (I know his father just got out of the hospital), or grumpy (she's going through a divorce).

Some people are private and don't like to share much about their personal life, while others tend to overshare. Each workplace also has its own culture about what is regarded as "normal" to share. It is important to respect the privacy of those who decline to share; just knowing that someone is a private person means that you know something about them.

We all share a commitment to patient care; it's likely that no one went into veterinary care for salary alone. We will do better when we can work together well as a team.

Sharing Personal Connections with Clients

If a staff member knows a client from outside of work, it should ideally be noted in the patient's record. This can help maintain a "small world" feel to a large client base, as it is likely that there are many connections between clients and staff. Mentioning the connection ("So, you are Chris's cousin!") can help a client feel relaxed and known by other staff members. In addition, it can help facilitate the animal's care, as a staff member can ask the connected individual for help interpret a client's story.

Start a Laugh Notebook to Share Humorous and Touching Stories

Clinics are full of humorous material, and laughter is a well-known tension and stress reliever. One idea is to have a Laugh Notebook in a common area where staff members can jot down funny stories, or to have one as a computer file. These should not be anything that would make fun of a client or that anyone would feel uncomfortable reading. Those light, funny moments that may pass all too quickly could then be preserved both for those staff members who weren't present and for anyone who might need a laugh at a later time. For instance, I recently saw a client who asked me to trim her dog's nails. She commented that she was trying to be better about doing it at home, and her system for remembering was to try to trim her dog's nails when she had her own nails done at the salon.

Case Story (Fiction): *The Effects of a Euthanasia*

Consider the case of a well-loved patient known to the entire clinic. Let's say it's a lovable cat named Cinnamon, an old diabetic cat who has been coming to the clinic for years and boards at the clinic to receive insulin injections when her owner is away. Lately, she's also been coming in frequently for subcutaneous fluids. Her owner is Dave, a friendly guy whose wife died of cancer a couple of years ago.

When the owner schedules her euthanasia, a receptionist takes the phone call. She's scheduled many appointments for Cinnamon over the years, but this will be the last. When Dave arrives with Cinnamon later that morning, the receptionist is the first person he sees. Dave is usually an upbeat person, but today he looks different; his face is tired and drawn. He signs the form the receptionist has printed out and takes care of the bill before the appointment. The receptionist marks the computer record as "deceased." Two phone lines are ringing as she blinks back tears and picks up the receiver.

The practice manager walks by to say hello to Dave and offer sympathy. They are neighbors. Dave frequently took Cinnamon out on short leash walks around the neighborhood and they always waved hello. The practice manager used to feed Cinnamon when Dave was away, before the cat became diabetic. The practice manager's mother was recently diagnosed with cancer, and she has often found herself thinking of Dave's late wife.

The veterinarian who owns the clinic noticed Cinnamon's name on the schedule earlier that morning. Dave and Cinnamon are one of her favorite client/patient teams. They used to see her as their primary veterinarian, but when Dave's schedule changed, he began to see her associate. She remembers Dave's wife well as they went to the same gym. She will make sure to speak to Dave before he leaves.

The technician goes to the clinic safe and removes the bottles of tranquilizer and euthanasia solution. They have already spoken to the doctor, so they know how much to draw up. They log them into the controlled substance book as they remember the numerous times they have given Cinnamon insulin when she was boarding. She was their favorite boarder. She always reminded them of their childhood cat, Silly Putty, who died at the same time of year it is now. Her loss suddenly seems very fresh.

The veterinary assistant prepares the room for the euthanasia procedure, carefully selecting a nice fluffy towel for Cinnamon to lie on. She remembers feeding Cinnamon and cleaning out her cage during her many clinic visits, and the way that Cinnamon would not let her close the cage door without a chin scratch and an accompanying purr. She is going to miss Cinnamon. After the procedure is over and Dave has gone, she will "bag" Cinnamon's body and give her chin one last scratch. Then, she will attach a tag to the bag and place it into the chest freezer in the basement.

The associate doctor hesitates before entering the room. He remembers his recent phone conversation with Dave and how Dave told him that Cinnamon was his wife's cat before his wife died of cancer. This will be an emotional visit, especially as Cinnamon has stopped eating due to a widespread cancer in her body. In the room, Dave at first tries to keep the moment light but breaks down and begins to sob after the injection has been given. The doctor tries to comfort him, knowing his words are inadequate and wishing he could think of something helpful to say. He stays with Dave for a few minutes, uncertain whether to leave the room just yet. Time seems to pass very slowly.

Clearly, the entire clinic staff is affected by Cinnamon's passing. However, there is no immediate opportunity for them to come together. The ebb and flow of the clinic is unpredictable, but there is always something to do. Each person is busy with their own tasks after the euthanasia: cleaning up the surgery area, answering the phones, treating hospitalized animals, visiting with a drug representative, and seeing an emergency that has just arrived. Each staff member may grieve alone even if it would help them to share their grief and know that others are also affected. Others may simply try to forget their grief, tamping down their emotions as they proceed with the next task.

Dealing with Dead Bodies

Those of us who work directly with animals, including veterinarians, veterinary technicians, and assistants, are faced with handling their bodies after they have died. It involves tasks not usually talked about, but which can affect us deeply. The listening for heart sounds, the removal of a collar. A final, tender touch conveying respect, affection, and even love. The removal of an intravenous catheter. The cradling of a head as a still-warm body is placed into a bag. The placement of the bag into a chest freezer; the body perhaps falling awkwardly if the bag is large and unwieldy. A wince as the freezer door is closed.

When I spoke to veterinary students about "bagging" bodies, they were eager to examine the topic; most had never discussed it before. Several had their own rituals surrounding patient bodies. One preferred to be alone in the room to fully focus on the task. Another tried to be especially gentle and tender with the body.

Veterinary staff may benefit from more reflection and discussion about the aftercare of deceased patients, and new employees should be appropriately trained before being left alone to handle these tasks.

Narrative Ideas for Clinic-Wide Wellness Care

Staff meetings can be a good place to discuss the implementation of clinic-wide wellness strategies, another is to have a notebook or "suggestion box" for ideas to discuss. Every clinic is different, and what makes sense at one clinic may not work at a different workplace.

One idea is to keep a quiet corner for anyone to go to when they need a moment alone or to take a deep breath and recenter themselves. This could be after a euthanasia. A writing notebook or some loose paper could be kept there for people to jot down their thoughts.

Dr. Ashley Emanuele of North Carolina says,

> When I was in clinical practice, I would let my staff members know if a beloved pet was going to be euthanized. With the owner's permission, they'd come in one at a time to say goodbye before we started the euthanasia. It provided closure for the team and the owners got to see exactly how beloved their pets were by our staff. It was always incredibly special. If someone felt strongly about being the one to be present/assist, or if they wanted to be the ones to make a paw print, we always allowed that too.

Some ideas for staff to grieve the loss of a patient (or client) together are to have a moment of silence at staff meeting, sign a communal sympathy card, and/or share a happy memory. A staff meeting could begin or end with a "celebration of life" portion as a list of names is read.

Suggestions for Reflection and Discussion

- Take a moment to consider what it would be like to hold a different role in the clinic setting. Write down your thoughts.
- How well do you understand the lives of your coworkers outside of work? Consider what you know about their pets, families, or hobbies.
- Think of what you can do to create wellness spaces or ideas in your workplace.
- How can staff members come together to grieve a loss they all share?

CHAPTER TEN

Diversity, Equity, and Inclusion (DEI)

Veterinary medicine is sorely lacking in diversity. Deprived of a diverse student body, teaching staff, and colleagues, many clinicians may be more practiced at dealing with diversity in our patients than our clients. Yet a large segment of the public owns pets, and to treat them effectively we need to be comfortable with narratives and world views quite different from our own. There are many kinds of diversity to consider, including economic, physical ability, mental ability, racial, ethnic, gender, sexual identity, neuroatypical, and differences in appearance.

Key Points

- The lack of diversity in veterinary schools and workplaces puts us at a disadvantage when caring for patients and interacting with clients and coworkers.
- To understand the stories of others, we need a sense of the diversity of life experiences.
- It is helpful to be aware of assumptions we may inadvertently make, for instance, about someone's ability to pay for treatment or seek a referral.
- There are simple and concrete actions practitioners and staff can take to increase our awareness and practice of diversity, equity, and inclusion.

State of the Profession

A 2013 article in *The Atlantic* named veterinary medicine the least diverse profession in the United States, according to data from the Bureau of Labor Statistics (Thompson 2013). Attention in the mainstream press has also included a 2014

DOI: 10.1201/9781003126133-13

article in the *Texas Tribune* that was picked up by the *New York Times* regarding the lack of Hispanics in the veterinary programs at Texas A & M (Maclaggan 2014), and a 2020 article in *Time* magazine stated,

> As more people of all races own pets, the U.S. Bureau of Labor Statistics (BLS) predicts jobs for vets and vet technicians will grow 16% by 2029. Nearly 65% of white households have pets, 61% of Hispanic households have pets, and almost 37% of Black households have pets, according to the most recent industry data. Yet pet lovers are faced with a predominantly white world once it's time to see a vet. Of the more than 104,000 veterinarians in the nation, nearly 90% are white, less than 2% are Hispanic and almost none are Black, according to 2019 BLS figures
>
> (Chan 2020)

The response has been a focus on increasing diversity within the profession. The Association of American Veterinary Medical Colleges (AAVMC) launched their DiVersity Matters initiative in 2005, seeking to diversify the applicant pool for veterinary schools. Veterinarians from the LGBTQ+ community and several other communities have formed groups with presences on social media. Some veterinary schools have begun to follow the medical school model of introducing classes in cultural competency; Texas A&M University College of Veterinary Medicine & Biomedical Sciences has introduced medical Spanish into the core curriculum for veterinary students (Tayce et al. 2016 Winter). The Royal College of Veterinary Surgeons maintains a Diversity & Inclusion Working Group (DIG), and the American Veterinary Medical Association (AVMA) has formed a commission with the AAVMC to promote diversity, equity, and inclusion (DEI).

These initiatives may simply not be enough, however, and in July 2020, several veterinary groups focused on DEI cosigned a letter to the AVMA to voice concerns and recommend action items (MCVMA.org 2020). One month later, JAVMA published a special report surveying veterinarians and students in the United States and the United Kingdom concluding that

> Comparatively high rates of suicidal ideation and suicide attempts among LGBTQ+ professionals and students and the relationship between climate variables and negative mental health outcomes suggested enhanced efforts are needed to improve the climates in veterinary workplaces and colleges.
>
> (Witte et al. 2020)

In November 2020, the AAVMC released a report examining selection bias from 2019 admissions data. The AAVMC newsletter summarized the findings by stating,

> admission offers were lower for candidates from underrepresented racial or ethnic groups, Pell Grant recipients, first-generation college students,

candidates from rural communities and candidates who aspired to practice in rural communities. Offers tended to be higher for candidates who were white, male, grew up in suburban communities, were not Pell Grant recipients and whose parents attended college.

(AAVMC Study Examines Bias in Admissions Processes, Standards 2021)

The report concludes that

the playing field is certainly not level for all candidates; candidates from disadvantaged groups must overcome disproportionate degrees of difficulty to achieve their goals...Whether or not the biases are intentional, the net effect of the various barriers is institutional racism, institutional classism (both socioeconomic and cultural), and institutional sexism. The results of this study strongly suggest a broad-based re-examination of our admissions processes is needed.

(Lloyd and Greenhill 2020)

In December 2020, the AVMA announced plans to launch a certificate program promoting inclusive workplaces (Mattson 2020a).

What is Cultural Competence?

Cultural competence, as defined on the CDC website, is

a set of congruent behaviors, attitudes, and policies that come together in a system, agency, or among professionals that enables effective work in cross-cultural situations. 'Culture' refers to integrated patterns of human behavior that include the language, thoughts, communications, actions, customs, beliefs, values, and institutions of racial, ethnic, religious, or social groups.

(CDC 2020)

Human medicine has developed several different models to teach cultural competency (Hobgood et al. 2006). The Center for Culturally Proficient Educational Practice describes a cultural continuum, originally introduced by Dr. James Mason, which is a helpful tool; movement along the continuum is described as representing a paradigmatic shift in thinking from holding the view of *tolerating diversity* to *transformative action for equity*.

The six points of the Continuum are:

- Cultural Destructiveness – seeking to eliminate vestiges of others' cultures.
- Cultural Incapacity – seeking to make the culture of others appear to be wrong.
- Cultural Blindness – unable or refusing to acknowledge the culture of others.
- Cultural Precompetence – being aware of what one doesn't know about working in diverse settings. Initial levels of awareness after which a person/ organization can move in positive, constructive direction or they can falter, stop and possibly regress.
- Cultural Competence – viewing one's personal and organizational work as an interactive arrangement in which the educator enters into diverse settings in a manner that is additive to cultures that are different from the educator.
- Cultural Proficiency – making the commitment to life-long learning for the purpose of being increasingly effective in serving the educational needs of cultural groups. Holding the vision of what can be and committing to assessments that serve as benchmarks on the road to student success.

(The Center For Culturally Proficient Educational Practice n.d.)

Cultural blindness is a common finding on the spectrum. People may mean well by claiming to be "color blind" but many groups and articles reject the "I don't see color" viewpoint as unhelpful, as it disregards or discounts both discrimination and the varying needs and differences of diverse populations. One of the best examples of cultural blindness is the "All Lives Matter" response to the "Black Lives Matter" movement. Yes, all lives do matter, but the response negates the lived experiences of a section of the population, as well as efforts to call attention to unfair treatment.

Case Story: *The Man in the Elevator and Cultural Incapacity*

My husband, Mike, and I were visiting family in Florida many years ago when we all decided to get Chinese takeout food one night for dinner. After driving to pick up our order, Mike and I got into the elevator with a large brown paper bag of delicious-smelling food. Another resident of the condo complex, an older man with a shock of white hair, got in with us.

"What do you have there?" he asked in a southern accent, pointing to our bag.

"Chinese food!" I replied, smiling.

"That's not *fooood*," he drawled, before the elevator doors opened and he walked out.

My husband and I turned to each other in stunned surprise. Had he *really* just said that? We were speechless. When we returned to the condo, my father knew exactly which neighbor we must have run into.

Although the brief interaction was well over a decade ago, and neither my husband nor I are Asian, we still talk about it. Along with our evening's supper, the man had casually insulted the food of a country of over a billion people. As evidenced on the spectrum above, his comment was an example of cultural incapacity. The man in the elevator lacked the capacity to even recognize the food of another ethnicity as food that he or his neighbors would consider eating.

Equity in Human Health Care

In human medicine, numerous studies have examined the disparities between clinical treatment for pain among different racial and ethnic groups (Meghani et al. 2012). In an article on the Association of American Medical Colleges (AAMC) website, Dr. Janice A. Sabin states,

> Racial and ethnic disparities in pain treatment are not intentional misdeeds: health care providers do not decide that some groups deserve pain relief while others should suffer. Instead, inequities are the product of complex influences, including implicit biases that care providers don't even know they have.
>
> (Sabin 2020)

Such statements should give all veterinarians and clinic workers pause. If people from certain racial or ethnic groups are unintentionally treated differently in a human health care setting, is it possible their pets are unintentionally treated differently by veterinary practitioners and staff? Could there be differences in client communication? In treatment recommendations? In the clinician's – or receptionist's – confidence in a client's description of their pet's level of pain or discomfort? Human medicine is addressing this problem in several ways, including education and ongoing research (Sabin 2020). Veterinary medicine also needs to be cognizant of this potential issue. Harvard University offers several free online implicit association tests (IATs) on numerous topics, including disability, transgender, race, skin tone, age, weight, and religion. These tests can provide a way for individuals to increase their awareness of their own implicit biases (Project Implicit at Harvard 2011).

Narrative Humility

Dr. Sayantani DasGupta, a physician who teaches at the narrative medicine program at Columbia, has coined the term narrative humility. Rather than believe it is possible to know the depth of another's experience, narrative humility opens us up to the likelihood that we cannot fully comprehend what it is like inside another's world.

> Narrative humility in medicine suggests that rather than looking out and learning all there is to know about racially marginalized or other communities, clinicians begin by looking inward and becoming aware of our own prejudices, expectations, and frames of listening
>
> (Charon 2017, 148)

DasGupta's reference to "looking out and learning" refers to cultural competency programming. While it is important to learn about diverse communities, it is not enough to memorize some statistics and "check" cultural competency off your list; to be truly committed to diversity is to seek awareness of our own biases and continually explore how we can recognize and overcome them.

Dr. Christina V. Tran, president of the Multicultural Veterinary Medical Association, explains there are many kinds of diversity; some are visible, such as race, and some are invisible or less visible, such as neurodiversity. If you exist in the majority of whatever category you are considering, she says, you may not have the perspective to understand a person's background, and even the terminology can feel foreign. Tran suggests that it is up to an individual to realize they could benefit from increased information about a certain type of diversity, and it should not be assumed that it is the marginalized person's responsibility to educate you about their difference (although they may choose to), as this puts additional pressure and work onto them.

While it is important to learn about diverse communities, it is not enough to memorize some statistics and "check" cultural competency off your list; to be truly committed to diversity is to seek awareness of our own biases and continually explore how we can recognize and overcome them.

Clients Need to Feel Safe to Share Their Stories

To treat our patients to the best of our abilities, we need access to their real stories and their real world. To tell their animal's story, a client must feel safe enough to speak openly and to be their authentic self. If a client keeps hidden some aspect of their lifestyle that pertains to their pet, we may miss or misunderstand important information to discuss about the pet's diagnosis or treatment. Doctors and staff need to be open to and comfortable with clients from different family settings, cultures, ability levels, and backgrounds to co-create a new narrative that works for that individual. If a client feels uncomfortable in the clinic, they may not return.

In addition, it is important to foster an atmosphere of acceptance and lack of judgment. Many clients confide in their veterinarian, and while we are not subject to the privacy laws of physicians, it is important to earn – and keep – the client's trust.

One example would be a gay or lesbian couple. Imagine a scenario where two men arrive with a sick dog. The record is only under one person's name, so the doctor assumes that the other person is a friend or brother and addresses only the "official owner." The co-owner feels uncomfortable and does not speak up about information vital to the animal's condition.

As another example, consider a pet owner with a conspicuous facial difference, perhaps a woman with a large port-wine stain covering her cheek or craniofacial asymmetry. Her cat has a chronic skin condition, and the practitioner dispenses medication and recommends a recheck. As she waits to check out, she hears staff members just out of sight talking and giggling about her appearance; they think she is still in the exam room. The recheck the following week is scheduled, but the client does not return.

To provide optimal patient care, it is our job to make sure that any biases or assumptions are left outside the clinic entrance to the best of our ability.

Implicit (Unconscious) Bias & Assumptions

Here are some possible assumptions veterinary practitioners and staff might make:

- This person is older, so he or she is probably forgetful or confused.
- This owner is young, so he or she is likely careless.
- Owners of certain breeds only have them for status.
- People who can only afford limited treatment won't pay their bills.
- Some women just have too many cats.
- Some men just don't know what's going on with their pets.
- This person looks poor and/or lives in a poor area, so they won't want to pursue expensive diagnostics, treatment, or referrals.
- This person looks wealthy and/or lives in a wealthy area, so they can afford whatever I recommend.
- This person is hearing impaired, so they can't understand what I'm saying anyway.

- This person doesn't speak English well, so they probably aren't that smart.
- We haven't seen this animal in 2 (or 5) years, so they must not be well cared for.
- This person declines vaccines, so they must not love their pet.
- This person looks different from me, so their values are probably different too.
- This person looks like me, so their values are probably a lot like mine.

We have all made assumptions. While it may be impossible to completely avoid them, we can work to minimize them as much as possible. The best way to begin is to mindfully cultivate an awareness of assumptions you commonly make. Once you have recognized an assumption, you can mindfully work to leave it at the door of the clinic or exam room and proceed with an open mind.

Clients with Different Abilities

Every practice should be prepared to treat the pets of clients with different abilities. Assumptions are important here as well; instead of picking up their cat carrier, ask the client directly if they would like assistance. Remember, some disabilities may not be visible, and never doubt a client who asks for assistance but "looks" healthy; many illnesses, including autoimmune diseases, can cause fatigue and muscular weakness.

An article in *Frontiers in Veterinary Science* provided the following recommendations about physical disabilities:

1. Always speak directly to the client (not to the helper, translator, or companion, if present), and maintain eye contact while speaking.
2. Ask before you help; offer help only if the client appears to need help. If the client does want help, ask how to assist before acting.
3. Similarly, if the client has an assistance dog with him, always ask before interacting with the dog in any way, particularly if the dog is actively working (e.g., in a harness, with the client holding the harness).
4. Be sensitive about making physical contact and avoid actions (such as grabbing the client's arm) that might put the client off balance. This caution extends to personal equipment such as wheelchairs, canes, and scooters, which are often considered part of personal space.
5. Don't make assumptions about the client's abilities or make decisions (about treatment options, for example) for them without their participation. Remember that a physical disability is not synonymous with a mental or cognitive disability, and the presence of one is not necessarily an indicator of the presence of the other. The client is the best judge of what she can or cannot accomplish.

(Grigg and Hart 2019)

Some disabilities are not physical, and a client who doesn't make eye contact may be dealing with anxiety or have a lack of social skills. Some people have difficulty reading nonverbal communication and may come across curt or abrupt although it is not their intention to be rude. This is often purely a reflection of their communication style and should not be taken personally.

Personal Pronoun Use

Dr. Dane Whitaker, president of the Pride Veterinary Medical Community (PrideVMC), advocates proactive personal pronoun use, that is, stating your pronouns (she/her/hers, he/him/his, they/them/theirs) when you introduce yourself to someone. I interviewed Dr. Whitaker, who recently wrote about Personal Pronouns for AAHA's *Trends* magazine. "The more that cisgender people use their pronouns, the more it normalizes their use and opens the door for conversation," Dr. Whitaker explained. He told me that when someone's appearance does not match society's expectations of male or female, it can lead to stress over being misidentified and/or judged. The proactive use of pronouns can relieve that stress by indicating a comfort level with different pronoun usage, which can make the client more comfortable discussing their animal's care with you. Dr. Whitaker suggests stating pronouns on nametags, websites, social media, and email signatures as well as when meeting new clients. Pride VMC offers pronoun stethoscope tags for purchase on their website.

In the AAHA article, Dr. Whitaker shared some of his personal story.

In the beginning of my gender transition, I was struggling with my identity and had to make some tough decisions on how my desire to pursue my authentic self would affect my career as a veterinarian. A colleague whom I greatly respected asked me how I would like to be referred to and what my personal pronouns were. I felt seen and heard in a way that I had never experienced before, especially in a professional context. Knowing that I had an ally who supported my desire to live authentically made me a better person and, in turn, a better veterinarian. Let's start to have these conversations about personal pronouns to help create this supportive and accepting culture, and to continue to make this profession a better place for all of us.

(Whitaker 2021)

Economic Diversity

Treating animals when their owners can't afford to pay for their care can be a frustrating problem for all involved. Dr. Michael Blackwell, chair of the Access to Veterinary Care Coalition (AVCC) and the Program for Pet Health Equity

(PPHE) and former assistant surgeon general, calls access to veterinary care "veterinary medicine's social justice issue" (Lewis 2020). In October 2020, the sixth International Veterinary Social Work Summit chose the theme, "Animals and Poverty: How It Impacts the Human–Animal Relationship" (Mattson 2020b).

Veterinary care for pets of people with limited financial means is sometimes considered a philosophical issue as well as a practical one. Some practitioners feel that pet ownership is a luxury, and individuals should not own animals unless they can pay for their care. For some clinicians, this view may result from experiences with sick patients and clients that cannot afford care, at times ending with the euthanasia of a treatable animal. This type of situation can expose practitioners to ethical and moral stress, which is explored in Chapter Thirteen.

Such situations provide an excellent example of the importance of keeping a "beginner's mind," as discussed in Chapter Three. When faced with a sick animal and a client with limited means, it is important to remember that we do not know the client's full story. We have not been in their shoes. What we *do* know is what's in front of us: a sick animal and (typically) a distraught, bonded human. The ethics we face are not whether a pet should be philosophically considered a luxury. Rather, it is how to best help an animal and person to the best of our ability despite financial constraints. While the situation may be challenging, it is important not to blame the client. People who face economic hardship love their pets as much as those with financial means.

And yes, there are a small number of people who take advantage, such as those who purchase purebred animals at high prices and subsequently seek low-cost neutering services. There are also those who loudly criticize the cost of veterinary care and claim that we should treat their pet for free "because we love animals." While these situations can be frustrating and hurtful, we should not assume that all clients who claim to have limited means are disingenuous and/or do not appreciate the value of veterinary care.

> The ethics we face are not whether a pet should be philosophically considered a luxury. Rather, it is how to best help an animal and person to the best of our ability despite financial constraints.

Innovative and Incremental Care

Tufts at Tech is an innovative Massachusetts nonprofit program that aligns a veterinary school with a technical high school to serve the pets of the local low-income population. Clients demonstrate need by providing an ID card for food or housing assistance. Veterinary students gain exposure to community care, and high school students gain the experience to graduate as an approved veterinary assistant (AVA). Tufts at Tech has served as a model for other programs (Lewis 2020).

The PPHE, based at the University of Tennessee, is developing AlignCare®, a One Health veterinary health care program that aligns connections with community resources to provide veterinary care to pets of low-income families (Program for Pet Health Equity n.d.). The program also promotes the model of "incremental care," which involves learning to prioritize tests instead of performing comprehensive workups, helping the client to best utilize their finances for the patient's benefit. The following is an excerpt from the Public Health Guide "Veterinarian's Role in Public Health."

> By finding compassionate ways to work within the owners' means and provide care, we serve more pets, defend public health, protect the human-animal bond, enhance community welfare, and reduce the number of pet relinquishments. We need to ensure our profession is serving more than just a fraction of society and work to remove the bias that exists regarding financial limitations. Learning how to practice "incremental care" is probably the most impactful way to work within a client's financial constraints. It is important to recognize the differences between gold-standard care, "the standard of care," and incremental care. Incremental care speaks to a spectrum of care options to fit within unique constraints. It serves as an important alternative to the animal not being able to receive any care at all. This style of doctoring is not new and requires using more judgment, more intuition, or empirical treatments to reduce associated diagnostic and treatment costs when the best recommendations are unobtainable. The owner must understand and consent to the fact that the treatment plan is limited; therefore, one must work closely with the owner to prioritize recommendations, communicate risks, and convey alternative plans if monitoring or limited treatment is unsuccessful. It is a tiered approach to patient management.
>
> (Brandstetter 2020)

It's important to remember that all veterinarians want the best for their patients, whether they practice using incremental care or are routinely able to provide "gold star care" to their patients and clients.

Case Story: *The Mystery of the Painful Jaw*

When I was first in practice, I saw a Doberman named Brody who had pain upon opening his mouth. I ran some bloodwork, which was normal, and sent the dog home with pain medication and antibiotics in case of an abscess, as the owner declined a further workup at that time.

Brody did improve on the antibiotics, but about a month later, he was back. This time, the pain was even worse. Brody's owner agreed to some radiographs of Brody's head. When I looked at them, I couldn't find anything abnormal, but I was concerned I might be missing something, especially as radiographs of the head are notoriously hard to interpret. I asked Brody's owner if I could send the radiographs out for interpretation. I also wanted to repeat the blood tests to see if anything had changed. The cost was roughly the same for the radiograph interpretation as for the bloodwork.

"Well, Doc, I can afford one of those things, but not both. You decide," said the dog's owner.

I was torn. I really wanted to see whether Brody's CBC had changed. But what if the bloodwork was the same? I'd be back where I started.

I chose the radiographs. The films were mailed out in a large manila envelope as we didn't yet have digital radiographs and emails.

Finally, I heard back from the radiologist. He had found a tiny area on the mandible that he thought was likely neoplasia. I began treatment with Prednisone, and Brody was able to eat again. Brody's owner was grateful I had managed to obtain a probable diagnosis given his limited finances.

I didn't realize it at the time, but Brody's case was an example of incremental care. The ability to rank diagnostics in order of importance requires the consideration of multiple factors. It may mean sending out targeted bloodwork requests instead of a full panel or waiting for the results of one test to come back before running another (assuming, of course, the animal is stable and comfortable). Providing incremental care can be challenging as it requires time, energy, and creative thinking, but it can also be intellectually stimulating and rewarding, and clients are often appreciative of their doctor's willingness and ability to help their pets despite financial limitations.

Gender Bias in Veterinary Medicine

In the not-so-distant past, women were actively discouraged or even barred from applying to veterinary schools. In the past few decades, this has changed dramatically, and women are now well represented in veterinary medicine and veterinary schools. Therefore, one might expect (and some believe) that a gender bias toward women veterinarians no longer exists. Sadly, this is not the case.

The gender wage gap is a very real phenomenon affecting women and their families. It has been demonstrated in a myriad of fields with numerous studies. Skeptics often point to the fact that women are more likely to work part time, yet the studies correct for hours worked. Women are seen by some as risky hires as they may leave or decrease their hours if they have children. Men, on the other hand, are viewed as more stable employees if they become fathers. The most telling factor in veterinary medicine is the fact that the AVMA consistently reports higher starting salaries for male new graduates when compared to female new graduates. New graduates have roughly the same skill set and experience, so in theory, there should be no difference in compensation. In 2016, the AVMA's new starting salary calculator tool initially instructed female respondents to subtract $2,400 to correct for the gender deficit they identified; the calculator was ultimately revised to provide clarification of the gender adjustment (Clarification regarding the New Graduate Starting Salary Calculator 2016). The AVMA's State of the Profession Report from 2020 concludes,

> As women continue to enter the profession, persistence of a gender pay gap poses issues for overall economic strength of the profession. This gap persists throughout careers, with mid-career practice owners at a $97,000 difference.
> (Bain et al. 2020)

Sexism is not solely about salary, and the gender wage gap may be more of a reflection of society's differing attitudes toward men and women than an example of sexism by veterinary employers. Women's work has simply been less valued than men's work in many cultures for generations and that value deficiency is reflected in the numbers assigned to salaries.

Ironically, authors of an article in Science Advances have identified what they term a paradox: "Those who think bias is no longer a problem may be most likely to express it." The article examines a randomized double-blind study of veterinarians in the United Kingdom, in which veterinary managers and employers were shown a performance review developed with the British Veterinary Association (BVA). The identical performance review was identified as belonging to either a male or female veterinarian. Reviewers who believed that discrimination against women was no longer an issue in veterinary medicine rated the female veterinarian less competent and the male more competent, and their salary recommendations involved a pay gap of 8%. Those who believed discrimination was still an issue rated the male and female candidates more similarly. The authors recommend applying their findings to other professions where women show increases in representation (Begeny et al. 2020).

One way to assess sexism in a society is to examine its stories. The Bechdel–Wallace test is a simple three-step test used to establish a baseline of female inclusion in films and other media. The test was introduced by artist Alison Bechdel in a comic strip in 1985, at the suggestion of her friend Liz Wallace (Merriam-Webster n.d.). Here are the criteria of the test:

1. There must be at least two named female characters in the movie.
2. These women must have a conversation.
3. The conversation must be about something other than a man.

Simple, right? Yet it's astonishing how many mainstream Hollywood movies fail the Bechdel–Wallace test. Conversely, if the test were reversed and applied to men instead of women, a movie that failed to meet the criteria might be termed a "chick flick" which would only appeal to female audiences.

Ten Easy Ways to Foster DEI

1. Visit the websites of the organizations listed below and follow them on social media.
2. Cultivate a clinic culture of tolerance, inclusion, and accessibility.
3. Check out the DEI CE programs on the AVMA's Axon CE platform.
4. Ask your local VMA to sponsor CE meetings about DEI.
5. Allow space for personal pronouns on new client and new employee forms.
6. Seek out diverse stories for your recreational time, whether reading or watching television or movies. Watch movies with subtitles, read books by diverse authors, view television shows about other countries. Check if stories pass the Bechdel–Wallace test.
7. Sample restaurant foods from other regions and consider exploring different countries and cultures on your vacations.
8. Check to see whether your local Veterinary Medical Association has a policy or statement on diversity. Request one if they don't.
9. Become familiar with local resources for clients with limited financial means.
10. List your pronouns on your website, social media, and client communications.

Resources & Organizations

Purdue University College of Veterinary Medicine offers an online Certificate Program in Diversity & Inclusion in Veterinary Medicine.

The AAVMC launched a free podcast series in 2015 entitled *Diversity & Inclusion on Air: Conversations about Diversity, Inclusion, & Veterinary Medicine*. The AAVMC also has free diversity & inclusion assessment tool worksheets for both organizations and meetings available on their website.

Here is a list of organizations that promote DEI in veterinary medicine.

- Association of Asian Veterinary Medical Professionals (AAVMP)
- Black DVM Network
- Latin x Veterinary Medical Association (LVMA)
- Multicultural Veterinary Medical Association (MCVMA)

- National Association for Black Veterinarians (NABV)
- Native American Veterinary Association (NAVA)
- Pride Veterinary Medical Community (PrideVMC)
- Pride Student Veterinary Medical Community (PrideSVMC)
- Veterinarians as One for an Inclusive Community for Empowerment (VOICE)
- Women's Veterinary Leadership Development Initiative (WVLDI)

Suggestions for Reflection and Discussion

- How aware were you about the lack of diversity in the veterinary profession?
- Write down a few more potential assumptions to add to the list provided in the chapter.
- Have you practiced incremental care, or seen it in action?
- Take one of more of the IATs through the Harvard University website to better understand your individual biases.
- Consider the last few movies you have seen. Did they pass the Bechdel–Wallace test? The reverse Bechdel–Wallace test?

CHAPTER ELEVEN

Veterinary Social Work

Veterinary social work is a new and growing field that exists at the intersection of veterinary medicine and social work. How can this new partnership between veterinarians and social workers contribute to the stories of our clients, our patients, and ourselves?

Key Points

- Veterinary social workers can assist our clients with difficult decisions surrounding euthanasia and difficult emotions such as grief and guilt.
- Veterinary social workers can assist practitioners and staff with their own wellness and resilience.
- Thinking about our own loss narratives can help us identify our own loss triggers, so we can best support our clients and patients.

Overview of Veterinary Social Work

Veterinary social work (VSW) began at the University of Tennessee, a school which has both a veterinary school and a social work school. The school's website describes VSW as "Attending to human needs at the intersection of veterinary and social work practice" and defines four separate areas of focus: compassion fatigue and conflict management, animal-related grief and bereavement, animal-assisted interventions, and the link between human and animal violence (Veterinary Social Work, The University of Tennessee Knoxville n.d.).

DOI: 10.1201/9781003126133-14

Benefits for Clients

Veterinarians are not social workers, although we have often been thrust into this role for our clients whether we were comfortable with it or not. We talk people through what may be some of the most difficult decisions of their lives. Some people may resent or dislike this role. And, we are not therapists. We are not trained to talk a person through their personal issues. However, that doesn't mean we can't address them. Fortunately, the field of VSW can not only provide us with referrals for clients who may be struggling but also help provide veterinarians with tools to better connect with the clients they assist.

Informing Clients about VSW

Eric Richman, MSW, LICSW, is the social worker at the Cummings School of Veterinary Medicine at Tufts University. He was the first veterinary social worker in New England as well as the first one at Tufts. Richman speaks to veterinary students to ensure that they will be comfortable bringing up a discussion with a client about speaking to a social worker. He explained that practitioners may be concerned about alienating or offending a client due to the stigma surrounding mental health and cautioned that some people may have preconceived ideas about talking to a mental health professional. Much depends upon the client's world view; an individual may have a positive view of talking to a therapist after having a previous relationship with one, or they may feel that such support indicates weakness, in which case it may be fine for "other people" but not something they would normally consider for themselves. Some may even have negative associations around the field of social work, equating it with the Department of Social Services or D.S.S., the agency that investigates claims of child abuse or neglect (Richman 2020).

When a veterinary social worker is on staff, such as at a teaching hospital, Richman says he introduces himself as a "team member who helps people talk through difficult decisions," initially avoiding the term "social work (Richman 2020)." For the many practitioners with no veterinary social worker on staff, initiating a conversation about the field may feel awkward. Yet the benefits to a client who does speak to a social worker can be profound. How to broach this delicate topic?

The first step is to have a veterinary social worker that you can refer to. If you don't know of any, you can refer clients to a Pet Loss Support Hotline as they may also make referrals to veterinary social workers.

Validating the client's emotions by assuring them that many other people feel that upset over their animal's illness can be helpful, as can Richman's strategy of emphasizing what you hope to have the person accomplish rather than the official job title of the person who can help them achieve that goal.

Another way to introduce the idea to a client is to utilize the self-disclosure method discussed in Chapter Five. In such situations, it could be helpful to mention that you have had other clients who have found it helpful to speak with a social worker. You might say the conversations helped ease their minds, alleviate their feelings of guilt, or manage their grief.

Even if a client does not contact a veterinary social worker or pet loss support hotline, your discussion of a referral may help them more than you know. For a grieving client, the simple knowledge that such resources exist can be a powerful validation for their emotions and can help them realize that they are not alone. It could also provide them with the comfort of knowing there is a "safety net" available to them even if they ultimately do not need or choose not to utilize it.

Social worker Simon Rochman recommends providing clients with a physical sheet of paper containing a list of resources and a heading such as "pet loss resources." Rochman explains,

> This will demonstrate to clients that you and your practice have put some real thought into considering how to help them. Handing the client that piece of paper with all of that information on it lets them know that you care as both a person and a veterinarian, there are others who are going through what the client is going through, and that the client doesn't have to go through it alone as there is support if the client wants it.

He also suggests checking with nearby mental health centers and hospitals with mental health programs to identify local resources, including pet loss support groups and therapists who specialize in pet loss (Rochman 2021).

Anticipatory Grief

The time to refer a client to a social worker may be some time before the animal's death is near according to Julia Gass, Veterinary Social Worker at Angell Animal Medical Center in Boston. Anticipatory Grief, also discussed in Chapter Eight, is the grieving that occurs when one is imagining the death of a loved one, who may not be near death at all. Just watching their arthritic dog slowly rise is enough to cause some people to contemplate their pet's eventual demise. Gass often sees both anxiety and hypervigilance among pet owners caring for sick animals, especially those that require a lot of nursing care at home. Gass recommends caregiver support groups for Anticipatory Grief as they can provide some much-needed validation from others in similar situations (Gass 2020).

After a Loss: Disenfranchised Grief and Guilt

VSW can play an important role after a pet has died, helping an individual or family to sort through the emotions of guilt and loss. This can be especially important as the grief over a beloved pet is often described as "disenfranchised," which means that it is not recognized by society. This can serve to increase the pain and loneliness experienced by clients. Veterinarians and staff work in an environment where most people take pet loss seriously, and even our family members who are not "animal people" likely acknowledge the importance of animals in our lives. Thus, although we can relate to the pain of loss, our own losses are less likely to be disenfranchised. Not everyone is as fortunate, however, and some clients may be in a situation where no one in their lives truly understands their pain or offers real support.

Benefits for Practitioners

The field of VSW is well positioned to help increase well-being among veterinarians and staff and to work to lower the high rate of suicide in the profession. Veterinary schools who employ veterinary social workers are helping their students to become comfortable with social worker interactions and to begin healthy self-care habits early in their careers. In a healthy clinic environment, everyone should be comfortable saying they may wish or need to speak with a therapist even if for just a few sessions. As social worker Simon Rochman says, "There should be no stigma in seeking help to handle the challenges of practice" (Rochman 2021). A few sessions with a therapist may help not only with the current problem but provide individualized coping skills to aid in dealing with future issues.

Clinics who have a veterinary social worker on staff may benefit from the social worker's ability to have end-of-life conversations with clients, freeing up doctors and staff to care for other patients (Cima 2020, June 15).

As social worker Simon Rochman says, "There should be no stigma in seeking help handle the challenges of practice" (Rochman 2021). A few sessions with a therapist may help not only with the current problem but provide individualized coping skills to aid in dealing with future issues.

Our Own Loss Narratives

Both Richman and Gass advocate for those in the veterinary field to explore their own unique narratives around death, loss, and grief (Gass 2020). Richman encourages veterinary students to create a "Loss Timeline" to think through their own experiences and reflect on their individual history (Richman 2020). The role of loss in our lives may directly affect the way we approach situations involving the death of our patients and conversations about euthanasia with our clients. While we cannot change our histories, we can acknowledge them as part of our own World View. An awareness of our own triggers and coping styles can help us support our clients and patients with minimal interference from our own past experiences. For instance, if a staff member was told as a child that their ailing pet "went to live on a farm" and did not have an authentic experience of their animal's loss, that person may be understandably upset to hear a client confess their plan to lie to their children. Having this realization ahead of time can help the individual to prepare for such an eventuality.

Case Story: *Memories of Monty,* by Julie Gass

Rachael is a certified veterinary technician in the Northeast who recently made a big move to her current position from a neighboring state in hopes of building her career. As a part of this plan, Rachael accepted a specialty position, an interest that was inspired by her care for her dog, Monty's, own health needs. Rachael was excited for this move, as it was an advancement in her career at a well-established animal hospital.

Rachael had been at her new position for only a month when her worst fears came true. One day, Monty wasn't feeling well and abruptly declined when she took him to the ER. While staff did everything they could to save him, Monty passed away in the hospital's CCU. This was devastating to Rachael, and as the days went by after his passing, she realized how difficult grieving for him would be.

One of the hardest challenges for Rachael was showing up to work every day in the building where her companion died. When Rachael would walk past the CCU, she would find her emotional response unbearable as she was triggered by the sight of it. Sensations and memories from that day would come back and overwhelm her to the point where she found she was avoiding that part of the building if possible.

Treating dogs of the same breed was also difficult for Rachael. She found that she could not bear seeing dogs that reminded her of her lost animal companion. She felt dread when bulldogs would be on the day's appointment list or when she'd run into one in the hospital lobby. Random encounters would overwhelm Rachael with grief, and she would find it difficult to focus on her job.

The days that followed Monty's death were isolating and difficult for Rachael at her new job. She worried that her new employers would regret hiring her and see her as incapable of doing her tasks. She kept her pain to herself and tried to put on a good face and prove that she can do her job well. She continued on with her work and tried her best to cope with the painful triggers of working at a new job where she experienced a shocking loss until she finally broke down crying in a meeting with her manager. Her manager, being sensitive to pet loss, approached her with compassion and understanding and referred her to the hospital's social worker for support.

During times when Rachael could not avoid painful reminders of her loss, she either made appointments or dropped by the social worker's office, where she had a safe space to not only process her grief but also feel comfortable being vulnerable and imperfect. While Rachael had a hard time with grieving for her lost pet, she almost just as much struggled with asking for help and revealing her vulnerability and imperfections. Once she did, however, her experience changed. It was still painful for her, but she was able to grieve without being isolated and burdened by the shame of imperfection.

Once Rachael started talking about her pain, her colleagues also opened up about their own animal losses and began sharing their stories of how they coped with grief on the job. This normalized what Rachael was going through, and she was able to feel more understood and less lonely. In a sense, she had an informal support group within her department.

Her colleagues rallied around her and took on the patient appointments that were triggering for her. Each morning, they would look at the appointments for the day and arrange their schedules, so Rachael did not have to take cases that involved bulldogs. Further, Rachael's colleagues would alert her when her dog's breed was in the lobby of the hospital, and she was able to navigate her day around those triggers for her grief.

The doctor in her department was also compassionate about helping Rachael through her grief. She made herself available to Rachael in several ways. One of the hardest parts of losing Monty was wondering if he suffered at the end and if there was something she could have done differently. The doctor went over Monty's chart with Rachael and talked through the medical details of what happened on his last day. She answered Rachael's questions and was able to break down the series of events that led to Monty's death in a way that reassured Rachael that he didn't suffer as she feared.

After receiving a compassionate response from the veterinarian in her department, Rachael felt comfortable talking to her about her work performance concerns. Since Monty passed away within her first month at her job, Rachael remained worried that she wasn't doing a good job due to her grief. Rachael brought her concerns to the doctor and was able to have an honest conversation about her fears, which were quickly put to rest. Her team's doctor reassured her that she was doing a great job and normalized how she felt.

While there was nothing in the world that would take away from the grief of losing an animal companion, Rachael's suffering was ameliorated by the compassion of her new coworkers. Rachael received support from several levels at her new organization. She received official support as a referral to the veterinary social worker, and she was unofficially supported with the efforts of her new colleagues who rallied around her.

> An awareness of our own triggers and coping styles can help us support our clients and patients with minimal interference from our own past experiences.

Compassion Fatigue & Moral Stress

Gass considers compassion fatigue among veterinary practitioners to be inevitable.

> "It waxes and wanes," she explains, "so it's important to pay attention to warning signs, because your body is telling you to take care of yourself. Everyone has their own unique warning signs: irritability, anxiety about going into work, depression, being overly tired, eating or sleeping more or less than usual, increased alcohol consumption – something altered in your own routine."

Gass advises trying to set aside time to take care of your own mental health, even scheduling a "mental health day" when such symptoms arise (Gass 2020).

Moral distress, according to Gass, is also prevalent in veterinary medicine, and our work is notable for the sheer volume of cases involving moral stress that we see.

Both these issues will be discussed further in Chapter Twelve.

Future of VSW

VSW is in its infancy, yet it has the potential to contribute greatly to animal caretakers and veterinary practitioners alike. Veterinary social workers can help alleviate some of the compassion fatigue experienced by practitioners and staff and work to devise strategies to improve mental health among all who work in the industry.

Richman feels that teaching hospitals are the most important area for VSW to make an impact as they can directly interface with students and expose them to healthy coping strategies. Ideally, Richman sees VSW as helping change the culture around mental health, normalizing discussions about mental health, and helping keep them as part of the dialogue, while also helping students practice and maintain healthy work-life balances from the very beginning of their careers (Richman 2020).

Currently, veterinary social workers are mainly employed by large veterinary referral centers or teaching hospitals. Yet their much-needed services could be utilized at "regular" smaller sized practices as well. One idea may be to consider the model used by traveling surgeons or ultrasound specialists; having a veterinary social worker rotate between clinics to spend half to one day per week at a practice, seeing both clients and staff. With the prevalence of Zoom and other telemedicine applications, a social worker may also be able to see individuals and/or run support groups via telemedicine.

Gass hopes to employ a type of therapy she utilized at her previous work doing hospice care and modify it for use in veterinary medicine. The practice is called Legacy Work or Dignity Therapy and involves honoring the life of a terminally ill individual by creating a book with photos, memories, and transcribed stories of the person's life, like an extended obituary record. The book then becomes a transitional object for the dying person, and finally a keepsake for the family members. For veterinary practice, such a book would be created by the caretakers, and Gass hopes that viewing photos and telling stories of the animal in their healthier days could help owners recognize and come to terms with their pet's declining quality of life (Gass 2020). For more on Legacy Work and Dignity Therapy, please see the Appendix.

Suggestions for Reflection and Discussion

- Think about how you would discuss VSW with a client experiencing anticipatory grief.
- What ideas do you have for the benefits VSW can bring to the veterinary profession?
- Consider the losses in your own life and sketch out a Loss Timeline using the one in the Appendix as an example.

Our Own Stories

CHAPTER TWELVE

Burnout and Fatigue

Narrative medicine can help practitioners as well as patients, by providing tools and strategies to help decrease burnout and compassion fatigue, minimize guilt, and manage distress.

> **Key Points**
>
> - Burnout can be decreased by emphasizing the unique stories of patients and clients rather than focusing solely on their medical conditions.
> - Compassion fatigue can be addressed by using narrative medicine to set emotional boundaries and recognize where our stories begin and those of our patients and clients end.
> - Working in close proximity to the distress and grief of others can be traumatizing.
> - Euthanasia and end-of-life discussions are unique to the veterinary profession, and their effects on practitioners can be profound.

Burnout

Sometimes, veterinary work can become tedious. It can feel as though we are doing the same things, day in and day out; treating the same conditions; making the same recommendations (which we realize may not be followed); and explaining the same information, over and over. Aside from reducing our work hours, what can be done?

Narrative medicine (NM) offers another way to look at practice. Yes, this may be the third otitis case you've seen this morning, but you can set your atten-

DOI: 10.1201/9781003126133-16

tion on the individuals, not the generalities. The animals are different, the people are different, and their *stories* are different. Rather than the third otitis case, the appointment is reframed to emphasize the interaction with the animal and person, with a focus on exchanging pleasantries, enjoying a narrative glimpse about their relationship, offering suggestions, and co-creating a new narrative with the client. Shifting your own narrative may allow you to appreciate the individuals you are caring for without concentrating on similarities in the medical cases.

If stories can function as an antidote to burnout, funny stories could help even more. Laughing releases endorphins, and funny stories can be shared with clients, staff, and families. Veterinary clinics are rife with humor and stories. In Chapter Nine, Narrative Medicine and the Workplace, we discussed keeping a clinic "Laugh Notebook" to keep track of those humorous anecdotes. Looking through the notebook during a break on a busy day could help revive tired spirits.

Case Story: *Flea Medication and the Holiday Dinner*

One December, I arrived at work to find a record indicating a client, Sarah, had brought her two cats to the emergency clinic the previous weekend after applying a canine-only flea preventative to them. The cats had both been tremoring but improved after hospitalization and treatment. I called Sarah to see how her cats were doing. Fortunately, they were recovering well, but she needed to schedule some follow-up care. As we talked, Sarah told me her story.

Sarah had been preparing a holiday meal for an extended family dinner when she noticed that both of her cats were scratching. Sarah immediately thought of her sister-in-law, who was due to arrive shortly and was not a "cat person." Sarah believed that this relative would be judgmental and complain that the cats had fleas. Dreading the criticism of her sister-in-law, Sarah hurriedly searched for some flea preventative, but all she could find was medication for her dog. As she didn't have time to run out to buy feline medication, she administered a small amount of the canine medication to each cat and continued preparing for the dinner. It was like a "shoving the dirty laundry into the closet before company arrives" decision. *I never would have done that if she hadn't been coming over,* Sarah confessed sheepishly. I told her that I understood how family could be. After all, most of us have a family member like Sarah's sister-in-law! Sarah paid heavily for her hasty decision, with both her worry over her cats and the bill for the emergency clinic and follow-up care. She would not make that mistake again.

The story helped me understand Sarah's decision. As a practitioner, it can be frustrating to see pet caretakers make careless and potentially dangerous decisions about their pet's care, and this frustration can contribute to burnout. Yet by coupling the problem to the "judgmental relative" narrative, it was easier to sympathize with the client and even see the humor in the situation, especially as the cats recovered well; I joked with Sarah that her sister-in-law should be responsible for the bill.

Treating Our Own Pets

When I was first in practice, I removed a cyst from my own dog. While everything within the surgery field looked the same as any other dog, it felt strange to glance away from the surgery site and see my own dog's familiar paws sticking out from under the drape. I decided not to do surgery on my own animals after that.

How do veterinarians care for our own animals? Some practitioners take everything in stride about their own animal's medical issues, while others find it hard to maintain objectivity. I have found it easier to have a trusted colleague become my animal's "primary care" veterinarian when they have a medical issue, or at least to have another colleague available to bounce things off and discuss.

Compassion Fatigue versus Empathy Fatigue

Commonly called compassion fatigue but also referred to as emotional or empathy fatigue, it is the specific type of exhaustion felt by caretakers who are invested in the well-being of their patients and clients. We've extended our emotions to an animal, a person, a situation – multiple times per day. But what, exactly, is going on here – how does this happen, and does it have to be this way? In this context, the words "compassion" and "empathy" have been used somewhat interchangeably, but this is beginning to change.

Recently, there has been more focus on exactly how our emotions are extended. Neuroscientists Dr. Olga Klimecki and Dr. Tania Singer have written about their findings using data from the field of social neuroscience, including studies of brain responses and neural substrates of empathy through functional MRIs. Here is an excerpt from their work.

There is a crucial distinction between empathy as opposed to compassion, empathic concern, and sympathy. Empathy refers to 'feeling with' – it involves vicariously sharing the same feeling with another person. The other forms of vicarious affective responses refer to 'feeling for' and are not necessarily isomorphic to the target's affective state. Empathizing with someone else's sadness implies that we also feel sad...Empathizing with others may also give rise to so-called feelings of *empathic* or *personal distress*.

...We propose that the term compassion fatigue is slightly misleading, since it suggests that caregivers are tired of feeling too much compassion, whereas the definition we use implies that the feeling of compassion should actually protect against burnout. Therefore, we argue that the term compassion fatigue should be replaced by *empathic distress fatigue*...instead of abstaining from empathic responses altogether, physicians and caregivers in general should aim at maintaining high levels of empathy and learn how to transform empathy into compassion and loving kindness before being trapped by empathic distress.

(Klimecki and Singer 2011)

In summary, according to the authors, what begins as a desire to help can go in one of two directions: toward compassion or "feeling for" or toward empathy or "feeling with." Continued empathic connection with clients and patients is both unsustainable and unhealthy. Compassion, while it may still take a toll, allows the individual to maintain their own boundaries and sense of self.

Dr. Bree Montana, program leader for Vets4Vets® (discussed in Chapter Thirteen), likes to use a metaphor about exercise and injury when she discusses compassion. "When you exercise, if you do it correctly, you may get microtears in your muscles, which then heal. But if you overdo it, and injure yourself, it can take longer to heal (Montana 2021)." This provides another way to consider the overextension of our available emotional resources.

Empathy Can Sneak Up on You

No one walks into an exam room assuming they are going to feel the client's emotions right along with them. While we expect to feel compassion, empathy can take us by surprise. The client reminds you of your grandparent or a good friend, you're tired or vulnerable that day, the animal is particularly friendly, the prognosis dire, the client shares a personal anecdote – and *boom*, you're not just extending compassion toward the client, you are feeling some of what they are feeling: you are *feeling with*.

In Chapter Four, we discussed entering the client's and patient's world. A clinician can become so involved in the client's narrative – and immersed in their world – that it can be difficult to separate from it.

The difference between compassion and empathy may need to be experienced to be understood, and it is likely that many of us will have the experience of over-empathizing with a client. If this does happen, we should remind ourselves that we must eventually exit their world for our own well-being.

Compassion Fatigue & Our Own Grief

Even if we avoid empathic distress, we may still encounter compassion fatigue. In a single day, we may give bad news, discuss quality of life, and provide euthanasia, sometimes more than once. Little time may exist between these episodes of extending compassion to others. Too often, we travel home, begin our evening responsibilities, go to bed, and wake up to begin another day without having a chance to process our thoughts and feelings about these experiences. One of the most difficult aspects of compassion fatigue is that it is not always recognized or discussed, and some of us have become so used to compassion fatigue that we think it's normal.

Working in close proximity to the grief of others can be overwhelming. And we are people, not machines. As individuals, we have own grief to bear: the loss of a loved one, whether human or animal, may be just under the surface in our own emotions. When people grieve, they may feel fragile or raw. While it is rarely done in our profession, it should be acceptable to ask a colleague to discuss and/or perform euthanasia if we are grieving a loss.

Many veterinarians are excellent at putting up walls while insisting we are fine, stuffing things away and throwing away the key. Yet this may not be the healthiest way to deal with grief. Consider how you would react if a colleague asked you to perform a euthanasia after recently losing a family member (human or animal). Would you agree? Most likely, you'd be honored to be asked and glad to help protect your colleague from preventable distress during their grief. Veterinarians grieving their own losses must allow themselves the time and space to grieve.

We grieve too when our patients die, and we should allow ourselves to experience this loss and feel the accompanying grief. As we grow into our careers, we may experience the loss of a patient we have known since it's youth. When faced with a bleak-looking lab report and an inappetent dog, we recall the frisky puppy chewing on our shoelaces and find it hard to believe that 10 or 12 years have passed. We may have grown fond of this patient and their family over the ensuing years, treating emergencies and health issues along the way. Now, we must advise them on final decision-making. The sympathy card we write may help us process our grief. Yet who will write a sympathy card for us?

Veterinary student Rachel Park worked as a technician before veterinary school. At the clinic where she worked, she was told not to exhibit any emotion during a euthanasia procedure.

"By putting others first," she observed, "it's almost as though we lose our own narrative."

This is emblematic of the need for veterinary well-being: many of us fail to recognize, much less prioritize, our own narratives, and thus our own needs go unmet. Over time, this can become an ingrained habit. Veterinary medicine must prioritize the ability of practitioners to maintain a healthy mindset while also taking care of pets and people.

Regarding euthanasia, most practitioners find that clients appreciate a small display of emotion surrounding a euthanasia procedure. There is nothing wrong with blinking back tears, reaching for a tissue, or speaking kindly about the animal. While the focus is not on ourselves and we must maintain the ability to do our jobs, many veterinarians consider the exhibition of some emotion a natural part of the euthanasia process.

It is normal to grieve the loss of our patients as well as the loss of the occasional client. Practicing mindfulness and acknowledging our grief can help us manage it, perhaps through a discussion with an understanding coworker, friend, or family member, reflective writing, allowing some time for self-care, or working with a therapist.

Social worker Simon Rochman points out that other losses can occur in the normal course of veterinary practice. "How about grieving when a particular client who you liked chooses to go to another veterinary clinic? You can grieve for this also. It isn't just death when these negative feelings show themselves in a practice setting" (Rochman 2021).

"By putting others first, it's almost as though we lose our own narrative." Rachel Park, veterinary student.

Euthanasia & End-of-Life Discussions

Euthanasia is unique to veterinary medicine. We cannot look to human medicine for guidance on coping with this particular stress and the swirl of conflicting emotions it may provoke.

> *I wish they'd listened to me earlier. Maybe I wasn't forceful enough.*
> *I'm really going to miss this dog; I remember when he was a puppy.*
> *I hope I said the right thing; I wish I could have helped the client more.*
> *For a minute there, I was back feeling the loss of my own sweet cat.*

Veterinarians are trained facilitators for euthanasia, the "good death." Most of us are fortunate to have support staff who are in the room with us, at our sides, who have our backs. Yet we hold the main role, and it is a lonely one. How many of us have heard repeatedly from clients: *I really wanted to be a veterinarian, but I knew I could never euthanize an animal.* It's an isolating feeling to be told that part of your job is unimaginable, undoable, and unthinkable. It can be all too easy to respond in kind, by *not* thinking about it, by doing it and blocking out the feelings, stuffing them away, even as we perform the procedure again and again. We may do it daily, even a few times on some days. It may be a scheduled appointment, or we may have little to no warning – the emergency, the appointment with the failing pet; it is something we must be prepared to do at a moment's notice. The clinic environment is a busy one, and we may not have an opportunity to discuss our thoughts and feelings with our coworkers even if we feel comfortable doing so. It can be difficult to take even a moment to pause and reflect upon the experience we have just had; to acknowledge to ourselves how upset the client was, our relief that the procedure went smoothly and our patient is no longer suffering, and our hope that our words of comfort were well received.

The act of euthanasia itself is not the only stressful part. For many, the discussions around the topic of euthanasia which can be even more difficult than euthanasia itself. A recent study showed that navigating a consultation regarding euthanasia decision-making was even more stressful than the euthanasia procedure itself (Matte et al. 2019).

Our Role: Professional Navigators

Dr. Harold C. McKenzie III, a professor at Virginia-Maryland College of Veterinary Medicine, tells his communications students that if they can navigate a client through the incredibly challenging euthanasia situation and the client thanks them when it's done, they have succeeded at a difficult task (McKenzie 2021).

We are the client's guide, not just for the euthanasia decision, but for how they *feel* about the decision. When our patient's heart stops beating, our responsibility to them ends. But what about our responsibility to the client? As we discussed in Chapter Eight, reassurance is extremely valuable to clients, and our words to them at that difficult time may be long remembered.

Does it Get Harder? Or Easier?

In 2015, Dr. Bruce Fogle, author of a textbook chapter on euthanasia and grieving, spoke to the U.K. newspaper *The Independent*. "As the years go by, it gets more difficult," he stated (Baggini 2015). This sentiment was echoed a few months later in an article in the *Washington Post* by Virginia Tech professor Dr. Harold McKenzie III, "It takes something out of you…it weighs on me. It's a cumulative toll. It weighs more heavily on me now than it did 20 years ago" (Shapiro 2015).

I kept thinking about that word, *cumulative*. It summed up my own feelings so well. For years, I had been doing in-home euthanasia as the only house call practitioner in my area. I had empathized with many of my clients, *feeling with them* in their homes, finding it hard to locate and reenter my own narrative. Perhaps for some of us, euthanasias are like heartbeats, and we have only so many to give. Or maybe the calibration of empathy-versus-compassion requires a certain type of energy, which may be more easily extended by some people than others.

Clearly, not every practitioner feels a cumulative toll from performing euthanasia. The same article in *The Independent* interviews Dr. Robin Hargreaves, senior vice-president of the British Veterinary Association.

> For Hargreaves, euthanising animals 'is one of the aspects of my job that I genuinely enjoy. It relieves more suffering than virtually anything else I ever do. I do more good by euthanising some animals than by trying to treat them.' One reason why he is positive about euthanasia is because he has reached a point in his career when he's seen animals die of everything, and hasn't yet seen one way to go that is 'anything like as nice for an animal as being put to sleep'…Hargreaves has an almost spiritual approach to this part of his work: 'We take a problem in the form of injury or disease that the animal cannot overcome and convert it into grief that the owner can, with time, conquer.'
>
> (Baggini 2015)

The past decade has seen a proliferation of veterinarians who perform in-home euthanasia as their main or sole occupation. It is likely the experience is different for different people and may even vary during different stages of practice. Perhaps future research will explore this topic. Meanwhile, we should be respectful of those who may hold differing views on the effects of euthanasia on practitioners and seek ways to continue discussing these effects.

The following case story was written by Dr. Éadaoin Redmond, a 2019 graduate who practices mainly on dog, cats, and horses. Dr. Redmond is from Ireland, studied in Warsaw, Poland, and is currently living and working in East Yorkshire in the United Kingdom.

Case Story: *Always Hurts A Bit*, A Poem by Dr. Éadaoin Redmond

"This won't hurt a bit," she said and mostly that was true.
A mix of white, fluorescent yellow,
A clear drip drip on the table.

"This won't hurt a bit," she said and for sure that was true.
Yellow now a mix with red,
Bruising hearts but silencing one.

"It didn't hurt a bit," she said as finally he lay still
Fur a flurry of clenched fists and faces wet,
Extended arm to all but her.

"This will only pinch a bit," she smiled, through forced chit-chat over wagging tails
Hours passing easily as if her hand had not played God.

"It always hurts a bit," she sighed to no one but herself.
His heart having ceased, yet hers heavy, guilty.
Unjust but always there.

(Reprinted with permission, copyright Dr. Éadaoin Redmond)

Dr. Redmond's poem beautifully captures the emotions which can surround euthanasia: the strangeness and loneliness of "playing God," the difficulty of moving on to "forced chit-chat," the grappling with undeserved guilt. I asked Dr. Redmond how she came to write the poem.

I chose to write the poem as I love poetry. I love language and how it has the ability to create an image in someone's mind of exactly what you're feeling without describing it in black and white. This is why I often refer to colour in my poem, it might not mean much to general member's of the public but my colleagues in vet med will understand the significance of the 'fluorescent yellow.'

On the day that I wrote it I was in a creative mood as I sometimes am and knew I wanted to write something. It wasn't a particularly tough day, in fact I think it was my day off and as far as I can remember no difficult euthanasias had happened recently but I knew I wanted to write about something I was passionate and emotional about so that the words could flow freely.

Dr. Redmond's poem opens a door to much-needed conversation about the difficulties and challenges some of us feel regarding euthanasia. This topic must be explored in both an open and ongoing manner, as performing euthanasia has the potential to profoundly affect veterinarians.

World Exit and the Overlapping Narratives Model

One way to appreciate the importance of disengaging from the narratives of others is with a visual reminder consisting of overlapping circles, like a Venn diagram. Imagine the "world" of every individual is represented by a circle. This "world" encompasses not only our physical presence but also our mental state and emotions. At different points during the day, your own circle may touch and even overlap those of many others: clients, patients, coworkers, family members. Many of these overlaps may be slight and superficial, but in the case of some of our interactions, they can be profound, and we may find it difficult to separate our own narratives from those of our patients and clients. These are the situations in which we find ourselves "feeling with" instead of "feeling for."

We can view a client and patient we have not yet encountered as separate circles from us. For simplicity, the client and patient are represented here by a single circle although you can certainly imagine them as individual circles.

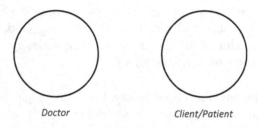

Doctor   Client/Patient

As we interact, the circles begin to overlap. During deeply intimate moments such as those surrounding euthanasia or the discussion of an extremely sick animal, there is the potential for them to overlap almost completely.

Let's imagine a story as an example. We'll consider a lethargic, anorexic, icteric geriatric cat named Grace, and an elderly owner named Frank, who come in to see their veterinarian, Dr. Fret. Grace is a sweet long-haired black cat who lives up to her name; despite her poor condition, she is friendly and purrs throughout her exam. As Dr. Fret discusses Grace's history with Frank, he senses the man's worry and concern, and as he views his patient, he recognizes the cat's weakness and discomfort. Dr. Fret is fully engaged: physically as he examines Grace and speaks to Frank, mentally as he considers possible options to discuss with his client, and emotionally as he recognizes the severity of the animal's condition. His circle touches up against and slightly overlaps with theirs.

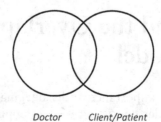

Doctor   Client/Patient

Frank describes a lack of finances, and although Dr. Fret discusses some options for workup and referral, he declines, electing to euthanasia the cat. Dr. Fret makes the necessary preparations, and shortly afterward he is ready to euthanize Grace. At that moment, Frank breaks down in tears. He explains to Dr. Fret that his wife died of Covid-19 after he first caught it from a friend. He was unable to be with her when she died, and he is grateful that he will be able to remain with Grace. Dr. Fret realizes that he is holding his own breath as he listens to Frank's story. He gives the injection and tries to comfort Frank. At that moment, their circles overlap nearly completely. While they are not the same individual, practitioner, patient, and client are exceptionally close physically, mentally, emotionally, and perhaps spiritually.

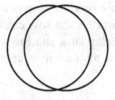

Doctor   Client/Patient

Eventually, the moment passes. Frank leaves the clinic, knowing he will return to collect Grace's ashes and place them next to his wife's. Dr. Fret wipes his eyes, washes his hands, and has a drink of water before turning his attention to his next appointment. Their circles have now separated.

At 3 a.m. the following morning, Dr. Fret awakens, feeling saddened. *Did I do enough to comfort Frank?* he wonders. Dr. Fret then reviews the entire interaction in his mind. With a jolt, he wonders whether he considered the option of treating Grace despite the lack of test results. *Did I discuss that with Frank?* he asks himself, taking a deep breath as he remembers that he did indeed discuss that option. Yet, the cat had been suffering, he reminds himself. Euthanasia *was* the best decision. Then, he recalls Frank's story about his wife. Dr. Fret feels again the emotions he felt in the exam room, and lies awake a while longer, lingering in the man's story.

The next morning, Dr. Fret thinks about Frank and Grace while he is stopped in traffic and while he is getting gas, imagining Frank waking up in an empty home, mourning both his wife and their cat. Although he is not physically near either the client or his patient, his thoughts and emotions are still with them. Dr. Fret is having difficulty separating himself from his experience with Frank and Grace. Hopefully, he will have time that day to write a heartfelt sympathy card, which may allow him to move on from his experience, recognizing what happened while allowing the intense emotions of those moments to remain in the past. While he may always remember Frank and Grace, he will hopefully be able to stop feeling as though he is still in the room with them and experiencing what he imagines are Frank's emotions, feeling the way that he would feel if he were in Frank's situation.

While many of us think about recent experiences and it can be healthy to reflect on them, it is also possible to overthink and dwell on them for too long. Thinking and feeling too much about another person's story is unhealthy. If our thoughts and emotions remain connected to another's circle for an extended period of time, it can indicate that we are having difficulty separating from their narrative and consequently may not be paying enough attention to our own narrative.

After an event occurs and we are thinking about it, our circle is interacting with a memory, or our imagination's version of events; we'll call that a shadow circle, as opposed to a circle in real time. A shadow circle should feel less and less "real" as the memory fades. The overlap of a shadow circle that does not fade, or that feels as though it follows us, is also an indication we may be overly involved in the narrative of another.

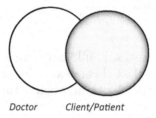

Doctor   Client/Patient

The narratives of our clients and patients are part of our own narratives. Ideally, they will integrate into our own stories, but not dominate them. Our own circles, our "worlds," deserve to be full and healthy, not overshadowed or minimized by the experiences and needs of others. The overlapping narrative visual can help us recognize we may need help separate from the story of another.

Another factor to consider is how often we find ourselves overlapped by a shadow narrative. Dr. Fret was awake at 3 a.m. thinking about his patient and client, and this happens to many practitioners. But how often does this occur? Is it rare, or does it happen weekly? Paying attention to the number of such incidents can be a way to help monitor ourselves for compassion fatigue.

Sometimes, just recognizing the problem of overlapping narratives may be enough to limit an unhealthy connection. At other times, we may need some assistance, such as speaking with a therapist, reflective writing, or self-care such as time off, meditation, or exercise. But the first step is to be aware this is a common occurrence in veterinary medicine, and to be mindful of its potential.

The narratives of our clients and patients are part of our own narratives. Ideally, they will integrate into our own stories, but not dominate them. Our own circles, our "worlds," deserve to be full and healthy, not overshadowed or minimized by the experiences and needs of others.

Boundaries: How Big Is Your Circle?

Now let's consider our own circles. In the above examples, all the circles were the same size. Yet there may be a lot of pressure on walls of our circle. We are caregivers, and for most of us, it is inevitable that at some point we are presented with more care than we can reasonably give, whether physically, mentally, and/or emotionally. There are times when we don't have a choice, as the animal is in the clinic. Sometimes, though, we may have a choice – the client who calls just before closing who could be sent to an emergency clinic. Much depends upon our individual workplace, but the culture of veterinary medicine is often the culture of never saying no, of always being available, whenever an animal is in need. After all, an emergency could walk through the front door at any moment.

If we never say no when it is reasonable to do so, we will not be in the habit of keeping our circles intact and fully sized. When we have not been able to maintain our boundaries, our circle can shrink, and when our circle is smaller than those around it, we may find ourselves even more vulnerable to the pressure from other circles.

To continue the circle metaphor, we will all come across clients who bully us, wanting to circumvent the systems we have put in place for our clients and staff. These people force their circles to be as large as possible and use them to push against the circles of others. Receptionists know these people well and are usually skilled at dealing with them. Those of us who interface with clients without a receptionist, whether for a house-call practice or emergencies, or who happen to find ourselves on the phone with a pushy client, are not always as competent. It is easier for many of us to protect others than to protect ourselves. And these "bully circles" know our weak areas. In addition, their bullying capacity may become further enhanced when they are legitimately anxious about a sick pet. Appropriate boundaries, therefore, are an essential part of self-care.

One common boundary issue is how clients address us. Common customs include "Dr. Lastname," "Dr. Firstname," and "Firstname." We are not alone in dealing with this boundary issue, and according to social worker Simon Rochman,

A major controversy in mental health practice is the boundary set by how the clinician is addressed by the client. Social workers almost always have the client call them by their first names. Psychiatrists and many psychologists, partially in terms of boundaries and partially to emphasize that they are the professionals, have clients call them by Dr. and the doctor's last name.

(Rochman 2021)

Boundaries

Dr. Sonja Olson, author of the forthcoming book *Creating Well-being and Building Resilience in the Veterinary Profession: A Call to Life* offers this advice about boundaries:

> How would you define boundaries in your own life? Do you have boundaries and are you prepared to explain and to defend them? These are guidelines, limits, rules for ourselves. We need to take the time to clarify them for ourselves and know how we will respond if someone steps outside of these limits. These are not necessarily rules for someone else to follow, but they do need to be aware of the 'rules' if they are to honor them. It is imperative that you are clear on what your boundaries are and implicitly and explicitly tell the world how you expect to be treated. Healthy boundaries are not harmful to others, nor are they by nature selfish, mean, or permanent. Boundaries are about personal accountability and are intended to be protective of you and of your energy/time/resources. Be prepared to assert and to adjust boundaries as you and as your life change.

Transforming Conflict and Reframing, by Dr. Sonja Olson

Conflict is a natural and integral part of our personal and professional lives. If we allow it to be, it can also be a formidable teacher. Conflict is an essential part of growth. The idea of conflict equating to failure is a false narrative. Did you know that in order for a tree to form heartwood (literally the core of its being), it must be subjected to wind? The push and pull, the bending and strain on the fibers, strengthen the core of the tree for all future growth. What a beautiful analogy to consider when you are faced with what the discomfort of conflict! The ability to transform conflict, to sit with the uncomfortable feelings, to emotionally regulate, and to set healthy boundaries are crucial components of well-being. Bring to mind and be true to your purpose, values, likes and dislikes. Of equal importance is to identify the negative self-talk and judgement that may arise in the face of conflict. Slowing down and investigating with curiosity the body sensations and the automatic thoughts that arise for you in the midst of conflict will provide the platform to move through the 'dis-stress' and shift from the reactionary amygdala and limbic systems into the 'upstairs brain,' the neocortex. These are moments of opportunity to not only practice mindfulness but for personal growth and fortification.

Suggestions for Reflection and Discussion

- Have you felt burnout? How have you responded?
- Think of times you have "felt with" versus "felt for." What were the differences? Has empathy ever snuck up on you?
- Consider your personal boundaries. What areas could use some help?
- Think of a time you have found it difficult to separate from another's story.
- How do you feel about treating your own pets?

CHAPTER THIRTEEN

Reflective Practice

Reflective practice is a fundamental way for practitioners to recognize and address the effects of our work on our own well-being. Narrative medicine gives us tools to incorporate healthy reflective habits into our lives, helping make our practice a source of satisfaction and pleasure. In this chapter, we examine how reflection can help practitioners thrive as well as prevent and handle burnout and fatigue.

Key Points

- Self-acceptance and self-compassion are necessary for optimum health and well-being.
- Mindfulness can help us observe our emotions, accept them as they are, apply self-compassion, and take action as needed.
- Perfectionism is common in veterinary professionals and can lead to feelings of guilt and shame.
- Self-disclosure can help us intentionally share our stories with our colleagues and coworkers to gain peer support.
- Dr. Charon's Parallel Charts allows us to practice reflective writing to process our own stories, as can the 55-word story model.

Reflection

What does it mean to reflect about something? Reflection is not about considering our own imperfections or mistakes and measuring ourselves against some internal standard. The goal of reflection, for our purposes, is to try to find perspective on our individual narratives, to put them in context, and to accept that we

DOI: 10.1201/9781003126133-17

cannot understand or know everything. It is to work on balancing our experiences with objectivity. Reflection is only meaningful and helpful in the presence of self-compassion, which is explored later in this chapter. Reflection is also best approached with a "beginner's mind," as discussed in Chapter Three, which is open to learning, as opposed to an "expert's mind" which may rely on assumptions and preformed conclusions.

Reflection is not about finding answers. It is about considering questions, and being comfortable with responses that are varied, shifting, or elusive. As discussed in Chapter Three, having a tolerance for ambiguity or TFA (also described as a tolerance for uncertainty) can be helpful in medical practice, and it can also be helpful when reflecting about medical practice. There are many times in our work when we do not know the answers and still must help guide clients to reach a decision and a new narrative. Naturally, as clinicians we prefer certainty, as do many clients, especially when it comes to end-of-life decisions. Yet not every client needs or can afford certainty. As Dr. Monica Mansfield, Chairperson of MVMA Wellness Committee (Massachusetts) and MVMA President-Elect wrote to me in an email,

> Part of the wisdom of our careers as veterinarians is that sometimes we have to go to bed without knowing the full answer, and sometimes it will feel uncomfortable for us...Our deepest client and animal compassion may indeed be to sit with that we are doing the best we can with the information we have and giving owners our best thoughts on the case.

We do not all need to become philosophers, but the ability to accept that some topics are uncomfortable, and some things cannot be known, and the contemplation of these issues is ongoing and universal, can be extremely helpful in veterinary practice. Mindfulness can help us try not to judge our feelings and experiences but accept them as they are. Ultimately, this can help us accept ourselves for who we are.

Reflection is especially useful for those who work with issues around death and dying that cannot be easily pinned down, described, or resolved. What happened to the presence of the animal that was in the room with us a moment ago and now is gone? How am I affected by what just happened? How does this shape my own understanding of mortality, and how comfortable am I with it after this experience?

Reflection can happen in many ways. It can happen through writing, whether journaling or writing poetry or corresponding with someone. It can happen through conversation, or through artwork, or just thinking while walking a dog, brushing a horse, or driving. It can happen through prayer or meditation. There is no "right" way to reflect upon something. There is only what works for you.

In a sense, the goal of reflection is to get to know ourselves.

Avoiding False Narratives about Ourselves

Narrative medicine (NM) provides several ways to help us recognize, decrease, and prevent compassion fatigue. These include the overlapping narratives model explored in the previous chapter as well as the techniques of self-compassionate reflection, small group reflection, and reflective writing, which will be discussed in this chapter. The use of Parallel Charts is discussed in Chapter Six as well as this chapter, and clinic-based wellness strategies in Chapter Nine.

Before we can consider these techniques, however, there is something we need to be aware of – the temptation to create a false narrative.

When it is tough to focus on or access our narratives, or if they are painful, it can be easier to create a false narrative about our own well-being. This is essentially a lie we tell ourselves; that all is okay when it really isn't, that we are handling everything well when we may appear to be – even to ourselves – but we aren't. Accepting a false narrative may involve forcing ourselves to accept that extra appointment when we really should have said no, suppressing a feeling of isolation, or denying the painful after-effects of delivering bad news or discussing quality of life with a long-term client.

Veterinary work is hard, not just physically and mentally, but emotionally and some might say, at times, spiritually. As tempting as it might be to maintain a coping strategy best described as, "It may be hard for others but not for me!" those who do so actually place themselves at a disadvantage. Maintaining a false narrative does not allow us to accept ourselves authentically for who we really are, which could hinder our performance and potentially lead to burnout. It is only by recognizing difficulties that we can address them, by implementing mitigation strategies and boundaries, developing healthy coping strategies, and recognizing when to seek support.

> As tempting as it might be to maintain a coping strategy best described as, "It may be hard for others but not for me!" those who do so actually place themselves at a disadvantage.

Self-acceptance and Self-compassion

Self-compassion is a critical aspect of practice which involves accepting yourself as a unique individual. Many of us compare ourselves to an imaginary, nonexistent "perfect" doctor. You may admire another veterinarian's practice style or consider them a "better" doctor: *Why can they convince people, but it seems so much harder for me? Why can't I remember those drug dosages? Why do I dread ophthalmology cases?*

We need to accept ourselves for who we are as unique individuals. This involves recognizing our own strengths and weaknesses, both as a veterinarian and as a person (Rochman 2021). This may also involve realizing that we may be different from an idealized future version of ourselves we may have held for many years. It takes a long time to become a veterinarian, which allows plenty of time to picture ourselves in our future career. For instance, you may have thought you'd enjoy surgery or emergency medicine, only to discover that you really prefer feline medicine or radiology and find emergency medicine too stressful. You may have always pictured yourself at a small rural practice only to find yourself preferring a large city hospital. It's okay. Accept yourself for who you are even if that person is different from who you thought you would be.

Self-compassion involves offering ourselves the same kindness and concern we would extend to a beloved friend or family member in our situation. A helpful exercise is to pretend someone else is telling you your own story. If your reaction would be significantly different to a close friend's story than to your own story, it's a clue you may be holding yourself to an unreasonable standard. Try to be as supportive to yourself as you would be to a trusted colleague.

Self-compassion is a growing area of focus for research. A 2019 study examined the results of a self-compassion scale developed by Dr. Kristin Neff given to 200 medical students. The scale includes questions regarding how we feel about ourselves and how well we care for ourselves. Self-compassion scores were positively correlated with engagement scores and negatively correlated with exhaustion scores, and the negative factor (self-criticism) was negatively correlated with engagement and positively correlated with exhaustion (Babenko and Guo 2019). Take the online self-compassion test to see your score at https://self-compassion. org/test-how-self-compassionate-you-are/.

In January 2021, the Center for Mindful Self-Compassion cohosted an online summit with talks from leaders in the field regarding the current research on compassion and self-compassion. During the summit, Dr. Neff explained that self-compassion is not narcissistic or self-pitying; instead, it involves including ourselves in a circle of compassion as an acknowledgment that we are part of a common humanity. As we share in the human condition, we should not exclude ourselves from receiving compassion; we are as deserving of it as anyone else. Practicing self-compassion, said Neff, is "humanizing yourself…otherwise you are dehumanizing yourself." Neff also discussed her Yin–Yang model of self-compassion. She described the Yin portion as soothing and nurturing. There is also a "fierce" side of self-compassion, the Yang side. This aspect allows us to act from a place of self-compassion to help protect ourselves, whether by saying "no," creating and maintaining healthy boundaries, standing up for ourselves and our rights, or not allowing ourselves to engage in harmful behaviors to soothe our pain.

Dr. Ronald Epstein writes, "Practicing self-compassion means neither avoiding negative thoughts nor overidentifying with them...Rather, you inquire deeply and respond with kindness, clarity, and resolve rather than blame, shame, or despair... it is a movement toward a healthy balance (Ronald Epstein 2017, 153)."

According to MBSR graduate Dr. Eileen Mulcahy, "Self-awareness is necessary for self-compassion, and self-compassion makes us more effective healers." Self-compassion, then, is not a luxury or indulgence only some can afford, but an important and necessary part of practice.

Practicing self-compassion, said Neff, is "humanizing yourself...otherwise you are dehumanizing yourself." Take the online self-compassion test to see your score at https://self-compassion.org/test-how-self-compassionate-you-are/.

Self-compassion Exercise

Try this simple self-compassion exercise. Picture yourself at a time in the past when things were difficult or painful for you. Now imagine yourself reaching out to your past self with compassion and love and giving yourself a virtual hug. This is done without judgment, and without trying to send a verbal message. It is simply offering unconditional compassion for your past self.

Mindfulness

How do we become compassionate toward ourselves? The first step is to foster an awareness of our own thoughts and reactions, and mindfulness is a pathway to self-awareness. Once you notice your reaction to a situation, you can then reflect upon it and consider whether it was helpful or harmful to your own well-being. The key to handling negative reactions is not denying their existence; it is recognizing them, accepting them, and applying self-compassion.

The first step is to acknowledge whatever issues are present. Being mindful of your emotions means recognizing and accepting them from an observer's viewpoint, without judging. This can be difficult because we may not want to feel that way, yet it is important to accept our emotions *as they are*. Once you have recognized an emotion, it is helpful to liberally apply self-compassion.

The order, then, looks like this:

1. OBSERVE your emotions as they are in that moment.
2. ACCEPT your emotions without denying or trying to change them.
3. APPLY self-compassion, as you would for a close friend or colleague.
4. PLAN as necessary.

That was a tough phone call, no wonder I'm feeling a bit frazzled. I'll just get a drink of water before I see the next patient.

I'm so tired today; perhaps I'll leave this phone call for tomorrow. It's really not urgent. I'll go to bed early tonight. It's been a rough week; maybe I'll use that gift card I've been holding onto and get some takeout for dinner.

I'm angry about the client not paying their bill after I did emergency surgery. Well, it makes sense that I'm angry. I think I'll talk this out with the practice manager when we have time and see if we can create a better policy.

I feel embarrassed that I missed that diagnosis and I'm mad at myself. I feel like I'm not a good doctor. But my boss missed it also and she said it happens sometimes. Maybe I should cut myself some slack. I'll talk to my school lab partner later; he told me he missed a diagnosis recently too.

Practicing yoga and meditation can help with mindfulness. The mindfulness-based stress reduction (MBSR) course is an 8-week course (also discussed in Chapter Two) which was created by Dr. Jon Kabat-Zinn at the University of Massachusetts in the 1970s. It is an excellent way to learn and practice mindful meditation.

> The key to handling negative reactions is not denying their existence; it is recognizing them, accepting them, and applying self-compassion.

Perfectionism, Imposter Syndrome, and Giftedness

Perfectionism is a common issue for veterinary students and veterinarians (Holden 2020) and can even contribute to a veterinary practitioner's susceptibility to moral stress (Crane et al. 2015). Imposter syndrome, defined as "the tendency to doubt one's abilities despite positive evidence to the contrary," according to a 2020 study published in *Veterinary Record*, was present in 68% of the 941 veterinarians studied, leading the study authors to conclude that "veterinarians in general have an alarmingly high prevalence of IS" (Kogan et al. 2020). A more general population study concluded that "clinicians and employers should be mindful of the prevalence of impostor syndrome among professional populations and take steps to assess for impostor feelings and common comorbidities" which can include depression and anxiety (Bravata et al. 2020).

Veterinary social worker Julie Gass of Angell Animal Medical Center in Boston sees both perfectionism and imposter syndrome as common issues among practitioners.

> I see many interns who feel that their value and worth are based on their performance. I remind them that no one is perfect, there are always going to be missteps, and it's important that they remember the successes and achievements that paved the way to where they are today, Gass said
>
> (Gass 2020)

Perfectionism can cause us to hold ourselves to impossibly high standards and to judge ourselves harshly when we fail to meet them. Perfectionism could also cause us to cling to a false narrative, as to acknowledge our real feelings would be to admit imperfection.

Many perfectionists hold only themselves to impossible standards, accepting imperfection in others and even extending compassion toward those around them who struggle to get things "right." However, some perfectionists hold others to the same rigid standards they set for themselves, and these people tend to be difficult to please. This type of perfection can stem from holding an "expert's view" as explored in Chapter Three and can lead to a habit of judgmental criticism. The "beginner's mind" perspective is better able to accept a range of different situations and circumstances and is compassionate rather than judgmental.

Another trait may link those prone to perfectionism and imposter syndrome: that of giftedness. Giftedness involves much more than having a higher-than-average intellectual ability; gifted individuals typically possess greater intensity and sensitivity and are often exacting perfectionists (Webb 2007). Although most of the work on giftedness to date has focused on children, there may be something veterinary medicine can learn from both current and future research on giftedness.

If someone were to study giftedness among veterinarians and veterinary students, they might describe many individuals as purposeful, driven, and intense. While these traits may have been encouraged and modeled in their childhood environments, the behaviors are typically innate, making them their own worst critics. They dislike asking for help or admitting weakness. From a young age many have felt different from those around them and struggled to find true, understanding peers. This may be a reason they are drawn to animals, feeling an intense connection. These individuals are often introverts with a low tolerance for superficial interactions, yet they can be extroverted when among true peers or during more authentic interactions.

Our Own Guilt and Shame: The "Guilty Aftertaste"

Our shame is often related to perfectionism, and we may need to remind ourselves repeatedly that death does not represent failure on our part, a problem we share with physicians (Laor-Maayany 2020). We may have wanted very badly to help that lovely animal and loving family. We may have truly tried our best. Yet we still wonder: could I have done more? What if I had thought of another medication, run bloodwork sooner, or tried harder to convince them to take him to a specialist? Shame researcher Dr. Brené Brown has a seven-word quote for just this situation: "Where perfectionism exists, shame is always lurking" (Brown 2010, 55).

Reviewing one's actions after the resolution of a complex situation can be helpful, but not if the primary reason is to denigrate oneself for any possible mistakes or items overlooked.

The main problem with our own guilt is it is often not recognized, and something invisible cannot be addressed. Many of us tend to not view it as a part of our story because we minimize its importance to our narrative, and we often overlook the significance and effects of our own feelings. There may be many other aspects to a particular story – the patient, test results, medication effects, staff concerns, as well as client factors such as emotions, compliance, and finances. Yet a narrative that leaves us with an aftertaste of guilt or shame should have Practitioner Guilt as one of the subtitles of the story. Once we learn to recognize guilt and shame, we will be better able to address them.

When We Make Mistakes

In my grandfather's time, there was no numerical system for keeping track of hospitalized patients. One day, there were two patients in the local hospital with the same name. One of them – a patient of my grandfather's partner – received a medication meant for the other, and it was fatal. Nowadays, there are far more checks and balances to prevent such accidents. However, they still happen, and medical errors are a major concern in human health care (Anderson and Abrahamson 2017).

In 2016, Dr. Marty Becker bravely disclosed in a *Veterinary Practice News* column about a mistake he made as a young practitioner in the 1980s. Not only had he overdosed a patient, leading to the patient's death, but he had also failed to tell the owner the truth (Becker 2016). Mistakes can and are bound to happen, and the profession would benefit from open discussions and stories about how to handle them both personally and professionally.

Physician and author Dr. Danielle Ofri recommends recognizing mistakes as a normal part of life. In a TEDMED talk in 2015, she stated, "Error is intrinsic to normal human functioning…We need to recalibrate our thinking to accept that errors are part of our normal human metabolism…. Our goal is to figure out how to live amongst our errors" (Ofri 2015).

How do we reconcile the knowledge that we have made a mistake with our sense of perfectionism? Perfectionism can make us feel worse by having us believe that if that one mistake is possible, anything is possible – it's all downhill from here. This could result in a practitioner's harsh self-criticism upon realizing even the tiniest of errors. Yet, we are all human, and we will all make mistakes. The important thing is that we learn from them, both by trying to not repeat the same mistake and by learning to forgive ourselves, as we are often our own most unforgiving critics. In addition, sharing these experiences humanizes us and the profession and can help others to know they are not alone.

Reflecting on "What Happened"

With a focus on self-compassion, it can be helpful to reflect upon our own experiences. Rather than suppress a bad feeling about an experience, take some unstructured time to think about what happened, and why it made you feel the way you do. Even if you wouldn't make any changes in your handling of the situation, just considering it with a mindful and observational viewpoint can help acknowledge your feelings and accept them.

As the following story illustrates, it is not necessary to understand everything about a situation or the inner workings of a client's world. Simply acknowledging that you got through a difficult situation can be helpful. As the story concludes,

> *Even after years of hindsight, I don't have this situation completely figured out. But, I learned the liberating lesson that there is no reason to get angry in these situations, because whatever the client is feeling is not about me.*

Case Story: *It's Not about Me,* by Dr. Lauren Bookbinder

One night while on emergency duty I admitted a horse with severe colic. All signs pointed toward a strangulating small intestinal lesion that would require surgical correction, and I was prepping the owner for the ultimate "surgery vs. euthanasia" talk through each stage of the exam. The owner had not been giving me a lot of verbal feedback, but did say that she'd had horses her whole life and had dealt with serious colic before, so when the time came, I thought she was well prepared for me to come full circle with the conversation.

I was very wrong. As soon as I started directly down the path of surgery, or euthanasia, she immediately focused on finances in an abrupt, aggressive way. I could see that the owner was very upset and emotional, but her words did not match her body language. The owner said that she wanted him put down and asked me how much of her money I had already spent just to tell her I had to kill her horse. I was shocked and angry. Didn't she know that I had been up for the last 24 hours dealing with numerous other emergencies, yet here I was give her what was left of my worn-out time and compassion in the middle of the night?!?!

Mustering some calm, I told the owner that I was very sorry for her loss and thought she was making the best decision for her horse. I informed her that we had spent $800–1000, which was the quote she was given over the phone for a standard colic workup. Euthanasia would bring her bill up to approximately $1000–1200. She was silent. I said I had some paperwork for her to sign and brought back our euthanasia consent form and estimate form with the $1000–1200 total. She signed the consent form and shoved the estimate back at me, refusing to sign an estimate that was over her initial phone estimate and had such a large range. Meanwhile, her horse is trembling with pain, my technicians are running around like mad, and my eyes are welling with tears – what was wrong with this woman?!?! *She* brought her horse to the hospital in the middle of the night, accepted our initial estimate, and now couldn't accept an additional $200 for the euthanasia? None of this made sense and I was irate.

I told the owner I was very sorry, but needed her to sign the estimate in order to proceed. She signaled me over into the other room and away from our students and technicians. For a split second I actually thought she was planning to hit me. Then, her face welled with tears. She told me that she lost her husband this week, and this had been his horse. She said she would pay her bill, but just couldn't sign that euthanasia estimate. I told her I was so sorry and couldn't imagine how hard this was for her. I asked if she could sign the original $800–1000 estimate. She agreed and hugged me. Then she said she couldn't see the horse again, left, and paid her bill in full the next day. Even after years of hindsight, I don't have this situation completely figured out. But, I learned the liberating lesson that there is no reason to get angry in these situations because whatever the client is feeling is *not about me* (Lauren Bookbinder 2021).

Ethical Dilemmas & Moral Stress

Ethical dilemmas may present some of the most challenging and stressful situations we will experience in our careers. There are many possible scenarios, and some are common: clients who won't follow recommendations to the detriment of their pet's health, clients who choose to euthanize a treatable animal, and clients who refuse to euthanize a suffering one. Our roles are complex, involving advocacy for the animal in question, but also an understanding of the client's (possibly the entire family's) world and emotions. We often find ourselves making recommendations based on incomplete information, whether from financial issues, a timing issue (awaiting test results, for instance), or a difficult diagnosis.

How are veterinarians affected by the moral stress we face? Unfortunately, we don't yet know the answer to this question. The following excerpt from a 2019 article in *Veterinary Record* entitled "Moral Distress in Veterinarians" informs us that

> Veterinarians are frequently exposed to morally conflicting situations, which often stem from conflicts of interest between clients, patient needs, professional duties and social expectations. However, moral distress in veterinarians has not been widely studied. There is correspondingly limited evidence to understand the relationships between moral distress, psychological outcomes, modifying factors, job satisfaction and attrition in veterinarians. Given the high levels of psychological distress they experience, investigating the effects of moral distress in veterinarians becomes imperative in the hope of improving their wellbeing. Further studies could include the development of a moral distress scale for veterinarians and evaluating the relationship between moral distress and job satisfaction, wellbeing and attrition in veterinarians.
>
> (Arbe Montoya 2019)

The following case story tells of a neglected dog; not the worst case of neglect I've seen, but a relatively common one. At times we may want to ask an animal's caretaker, *how did you let it get this bad?*

Case Story: *The Man Who Had Fallen Upon Hard Times*

As I looked at the record, I noticed it had been over 2 years since we had seen this little Cockapoo named Kahlua. My first impression of the dog was that he was terribly matted. His owner, who had arrived in the exam room with a child and an infant in a carrier, said he needed Kahlua's vaccinations to be updated due to a grooming appointment scheduled for the following week. I was relieved to hear a grooming had already been scheduled, as the dog looked like a "before" picture from an animal rescue association.

"I know he looks bad," the man admitted before I could say anything. "We fell upon some hard times. But we're doing better now," he said, turning to smile at the children.

I assured him we would get Kahlua up to date.

As I examined the dog, I realized just how matted he was. I could barely find his ears or auscult his heart, and the fur matted to his legs made the blood draw difficult. After I finished the exam and vaccination update, I looked at the schedule. I had a few minutes, so I told the man I would take Kahlua out back to the treatment area and shave a few matts to hold him over until his grooming appointment. I just couldn't let the animal walk out of the clinic in that condition.

Out back, my assistant Michelle held Kahlua as I picked up an ear. The groomer was going to have her hands full with this one, we commented. I winced as I worked on a large matt that extended all the way down Kahlua's neck. When I finished, I realized the matt had been restricting the dog's ability to turn his head. With his newfound mobility, Kahlua tossed his head and began to resist being restrained, so I stopped shaving. Out of earshot of the dog's family, Michelle and I shared some choice words about his condition.

As I walked back to the exam room, I felt conflicting emotions. On the one hand, the dog's caretaker had demonstrated concern for him, regretting his inability to care for his pet and wanted him to be comfortable. On the other hand, the dog had been neglected to the point of chronic discomfort. Part of me wanted to yell at the man, even though that wasn't my typical behavior. Yet he had brought his dog into the clinic; if I made him feel bad, he may not bring his dog for future veterinary care. I wanted the man to be aware of his dog's needs going forward, which was more important than emphasizing the damage already done. It was up to me to advocate on Kahlua's behalf; I needed to walk a line between criticizing his care of his dog and emphasizing the importance of grooming for his dog's quality of life.

Ultimately, I smiled at the man and explained how the matts had restricted Kahlua's ability to turn his head. I recommended he be groomed regularly and shaved down if it was difficult to have him groomed often. The man smiled and agreed.

As they left, I wondered: had I been forceful enough? Could another veterinarian have done better?

The moral stress I had experienced caused me to experience several emotions, including frustration and self-doubt. Yet, these types of situations are not uncommon in general practice. Veterinary medicine could be helped by an increased awareness of the realities of moral stress, and reflection can help clinicians appreciate the difficulties of such situations and realize that we are not alone.

Self-disclosure: Sharing Our Stories with Colleagues and Coworkers

In Chapter Five, Making a Plan, we discussed self-disclosure to clients, both in terms of our experiences as a pet owner and as a clinician, sharing stories with clients about other patients you've worked with. But what about the issue of self-disclosure with our own colleagues and coworkers? Can we share our deeper stories with our peers?

Ideally, we should be able to both celebrate our successes and acknowledge our perceived failures with our coworkers. However, many of us find it difficult to truly share our concerns with others. As a result, in the words of Dr. Launer, "clinical anecdotes may be exchanged more as tokens of bravado than as requests for support" (Launer 2002, 104). Raise your hand if you have done this! Dr. Launer concludes there are not enough opportunities for primary care practitioners to discuss and reflect upon difficult cases and notes that some aspects of practice have a "macho" culture (Launer 2002, 104). As a result, a veterinarian's lack of sleep as she worries over a case could be cleverly disguised as a casual remark to a colleague the following day, thinking if it progresses further into a conversation about the case, it would be nice, but if not, it could pass as a casual comment.

Both self-disclosure conversations and discussions about the health of our pet or that of a coworker should not be reduced to what Dr. Annie Wayne, assistant professor at Cummings School of Veterinary Medicine at Tufts University, refers to as "hallway conversations." Real, focused self-disclosure should ideally happen when there are no distractions and low likelihood of interruptions, perhaps in a small group setting. Self-disclosure is not a substitute for therapy, and if someone is continually struggling, a visit with a therapist or veterinary social worker may be beneficial.

The Small Group Model

The value of sharing clinical experiences with small groups of colleagues has been known for many years. In the 1950s, British psychoanalysts Michael and Enid Balint invented the idea of a small group format for physicians to discuss cases with a focus on the doctor–patient relationship (Yazdankhahfard et al. 2019). The idea caught on, and there are now Balint societies in several countries, including the United States, the United Kingdom, and Australia/New Zealand. Balint groups have been accepted as assisting with compassion fatigue and burnout in practicing physicians (Benson and Magraith 2005), as well as playing a role in medical student education (Torppa et al. 2008).

NM has borrowed from the Balint model in that facilitated small groups are utilized in NM workshops and facilitator training sessions. In my experience teaching NM as an elective for students at the Cummings School of Veterinary Medicine at Tufts University, I have witnessed the positive impact of a small, facilitated group. While sharing a safe space with a handful of colleagues, it is possible to reflect upon common situations in veterinary medicine that are not often explored. Small group discussions also provide a sense of community regarding issues that may be difficult to discuss.

Groups I attended and facilitated met virtually due to the pandemic, and virtual groups may be a model to consider for veterinarians and veterinary students in the future. Students could continue a relationship with classmates after graduation, meeting once a month to discuss the realities of practice, or form new groups with peers in similar practice situations.

Such small group sessions would not be group therapy sessions, and ideally would be facilitated, which may be difficult to maintain. One idea would be for participants to take turns facilitating after completing a training session. Perhaps the field of veterinary social work could assist with the development of such a model.

Dr. Charon's Parallel Chart and Discussion Groups

In Chapter Six, we explored keeping a "Parallel Chart" in addition to the official patient record. Writing in parallel with the patient's official medical chart can be a helpful way to reflect upon experiences with a client and patient. The writer is allowed free rein to describe their personal thoughts and experiences. This chart does not have to be read by anyone, although it can be helpful to share it, especially in the facilitated small group model preferred by Dr. Charon, who writes that her students "have found comfort in hearing one another read Parallel Chart entries, commenting often that they no longer feel alone in their mournfulness or sadness or guilt" (Charon 2006, 156).

Dr. Charon distinguishes her Parallel Chart discussion groups from support groups or group therapy and feels that they should be considered a regular part of medical student training to increase the capacity for "effective clinical work." She points out that she is not a mental health professional and has not been trained to run group therapy sessions. Rather, she is a close reader and listener who explores the narratives with her students, encouraging them to respond to what they see, what they hear, and what they would like to learn more about (Charon 2006, 156–159).

Reflective Writing

Reflective writing can be a pathway toward a better understanding of ourselves (Charon 2006, 139). When writing, try to free associate and not overplan. Remember this is only a rough draft to get your thoughts down as soon as they arise. If you are focused on creating a polished document, your writing is likely to be more stilted and less creative.

Here are some things to consider after you have written something:

- How did you feel *while* you were writing? Maybe you felt focused, maybe you were tired or frustrated. It doesn't matter. Just recognize and accept how you felt.
- How did you feel when you read it afterward? Again, no judgment on how you felt. Maybe you were disappointed or irritated, maybe you were excited and pleased by what you'd written. Maybe you didn't have much of a reaction at all. It's all okay, just notice it.
- Did it make you realize anything you hadn't thought of before? Sometimes, just the act of writing can cause us to examine a situation in another way and help us reach a different perspective. It can also help create a sense of focus to help work through thoughts or emotions you didn't realize at the time.
- Did anything surprise you? Did you learn anything about how you felt that you weren't aware of before you started writing, or before you *thought* about writing about this subject?
- Have you written this way before (journals, emails, letters)? People used to write letters as a main means of communication, but this is far less common now. Think about times you may have written this way before and how this experience compares.

Try not to compare your writing to other things you may have written. Don't worry about doing it wrong; you're not. In the same way, try not to concern yourself with what other people may be writing about. It's also okay to take "reflection breaks" as you write to think about any feelings or thoughts the writing has brought to the surface. But don't stop for too long. If there's something you'd like to remember for later, jot it down.

As you continue with reflective writing, try to mix things up a bit; if you are used to typing on a computer, try writing freehand and see if it feels different to you. Try writing in different places – at a table, on the sofa, outside if possible.

Carry a small notebook with you, or even a scrap of paper in your pocket, to write down anything that happens during the day that you may want to write about later, when you have time.

Good things to write about are ideas that are "sticky" – encounters or thoughts that keep coming up in your mind. *Why did she say that? What did he mean? Why did I do that? I feel like I could have done more.*

The 55-Word Story

Marcia Day Childress, PhD, directs the programs in humanities in the Center for Health Humanities and Ethics at the University of Virginia, where she teaches reflective writing to medical students. Dr. Childress encourages the use of a writing tool called "The 55-word story" which has been described in *JAMA* (Christianson 2002). An article she authored in the *AMA Journal of Ethics* beautifully describes this brief form of literary reflection.

> As a literary form, it is simple. As an assignment, it may or may not be written to a prompt. As a task, it is blessedly brief—also game-like, distractingly, even addictively, so. Here is the trick: the story must be *55 words exactly*, no more and no fewer (not counting an optional title). There are no other rules. The exercise involves words and numbers, composing and counting—a lively combination of mental functions. The story may be written fast (in under ten minutes) or slow (take a week); it need not use complete sentences; it may be arranged on the page any which way; its word count may be edited down or built up to the magic 55; in topic and tone it may be dark or droll, silly, sweet, or stunning. Perhaps most importantly, anyone can write a 55-word story. Also, in my experience, more doctors than not love this exercise and many make it a permanent addition to their medical toolkit.
>
> (Childress 2017)

The 55-word story has great potential for veterinary medicine as a brief format for narrative reflection. The short length makes it less intimidating than facing a large blank piece of paper or screen and planning to fill it with words. And if the story does spark a well of creative writing, it can always be lengthened.

Vets4Vets®

Vets4Vets® is a resource of the VIN Foundation, a nonprofit providing helpful support to preveterinary students, veterinary students, and veterinarians at no cost, started by the veterinary information network (VIN) in 2005. Vets4Vets® is a free resource that is available to all veterinary students and veterinarians, not just VIN members. Among the resources offered are one-on-one peer-to-peer support, weekly support groups, remote mentoring, student debt assistance, as well as groups for veterinarians in recovery and those dealing with cancer.

Dr. Bree Montana, Vets4Vets® Program Leader, says that one thing she hears repeatedly from veterinarians who contact the program is the statement, *I feel so much better just knowing that I'm not alone.*

"All of us are so much more alike than we are different," Dr. Montana said (Montana 2021).

Self-care: Creating Your Own Wellness Toolbox

Much focus has been placed, rightly, on self-care in our profession. Veterinary work is hard, and no one is exempt. As part of our own narratives, we can individualize our strategies for self-care. We can each create a virtual toolbox of self-care ideas and activities, so once we are good at recognizing when we could use self-care, we have some ideas already thought out and ready to go. This can also prevent us from turning to counterproductive or unhealthy ways to react when we are having a difficult time.

Veterinary Self-care Toolbox Template:

- Ideas for favorite food, whether cookies or sushi
- Candy or chocolate
- Reflective writing is a free activity discussed in previous section
- Exercise is beneficial for self-care, write down three forms of exercise, i.e., walking dog, Yoga, Tai Chi
- Meditation
- Getting into nature
- Going for a walk or a drive
- Mental escape – read a book, watch a movie, or binge-watch a favorite show
- Creative activity – drawing, singing, writing, cooking
- Connection – talk to a friend or family member, possibly someone you haven't connected with in a while
- Physical – take a hot bath, get a massage
- Buy yourself a present – pretend you are gift shopping for yourself. Give yourself a budget and splurge on something you might gift a friend. Even a few dollars could get you a gourmet candy bar, fancy coffee, or a magazine. Or, take that gift card hiding in a drawer and put it to use.
- Allow yourself to wallow – set a timer for 5 or 10 minutes and indulge your self-pity with a world-class wallow before intentionally putting your thoughts away and moving on to another self-care activity.

- Music – list some music that can help you relax (Classical, Jazz), pep you up (80's music, *Hamilton* soundtrack), or will reflect your mood (Pink Floyd).
- Laugh – read some comics or jokes, watch funny videos or your favorite comedy movie.

You can also make yourself a physical toolbox, with self-care items such as:

- A nice notebook and pen to write your thoughts
- A gift card leftover from a birthday or holiday
- A thank you card from a client, to remember how you made a positive difference for someone
- A scented candle
- A joke book to make you laugh

Suggestions for Reflection and Discussion

- Write reflectively about a time when you had a hard time separating from another individual's narrative.
- Take the self-compassion test online. What did you learn from the results?
- The author of the study on moral distress in veterinarians mentioned creating a moral distress scale. How would you go about creating such a scale?
- Have you ever created a false narrative about your reaction to a situation?
- Write a 55-word story about self-disclosure.

CHAPTER FOURTEEN

Moving Forward

The formal practice of narrative medicine is in its infancy for both human medicine and in veterinary medicine. We are at the forefront of a new approach, one that combines the best of "old-school" practices with cutting-edge perspectives, ideas, and collaborations.

Where do we go from here?

Key Points

- Multiple narrative medicine (NM) perspectives exist in human medicine, and there is room for many in veterinary medicine as well.
- A focus on NM can begin before veterinary school, and admission requirements could better reflect the real needs of practicing veterinarians.
- The pandemic may offer us different ways to think about veterinary practice.
- By sharing our stories, we help one another as well as ourselves.

A Request for Case Stories & Veterinary Narratives

Case studies are commonly used in veterinary training and continuing education. In this book, I have chosen to refer to examples as case stories rather than studies. Many people find stories or anecdotes easier to remember than a list of details and test results. Linking an example to a story or a funny anecdote can be a helpful way to get students to better retain material.

DOI: 10.1201/9781003126133-18

The Connection Triangle is often a good focus for a story. Photos for case stories could include the client as well as the patient, so viewers could observe the human–animal bond between the individuals.

Veterinary narratives can take many forms – stories, poems, photographs, paintings, and other representations of our work. They may relate to our work directly or indirectly to provide a format to reflect upon and discuss some of the many themes we deal within our work, including love and loss.

A Narrative Focus Before Veterinary School

Different veterinary schools may have different entrance requirements, but most are heavy on the "hard sciences" such as physics, chemistry, organic chemistry, and biology. While some courses are essential to the study of veterinary medicine, others may be required more as "weeder" classes due to their difficulty than their actual relevance to veterinary practice. In addition, there are many areas of study which are not traditionally required yet could prove extremely useful. It may be time to reevaluate prerequisite courses for veterinary school admission. Similar recommendations are also being made for medical students (Swede and Marci 2016). Required courses could still be rigorous while being more relevant to both veterinary school and veterinary medical practice.

Two semesters of both physics and organic chemistry, each with labs, may not actually be useful for most veterinary practitioners. However, an introductory class in psychology could be indispensable, both as an introduction to veterinary behavior issues and to gain an understanding of client (and coworker) behavior. A class in sociology or psychology that discusses grieving, including the work of Elisabeth Kubler-Ross on the steps of the grieving process, should be required, as unless we treat primarily long-lived species such as parrots or sea turtles, veterinarians are likely to outlive the vast majority of our patients, and our clients are likely to outlive most of their pets. A certain degree of comfort and familiarity around the issues of grief and death are essential for most veterinarians. A class in philosophy and/or ethics could introduce habits of reflection, as could courses in literature and humanities.

When I put the question of undergraduate requirements to a group of veterinary students, they had several excellent suggestions. Kayla Blyton had taken a course in positive psychology which she felt helped her build resilience, an important skill in veterinary practice. Lauren Fay felt that a public speaking course would be valuable, and Elina Grunkina suggested statistics as a requirement instead of calculus, as well as a business class.

Courses could also be encouraged which foster creativity and curiosity, such as art appreciation and literature courses. In addition, if undergraduate requirements allowed and encouraged pre-veterinary students to partake of junior year abroad programs (which are often discouraged due to the rigorous curriculum), students may accumulate experiences which could contribute to a knowledge of and appreciation for cultural diversity.

Narrative Medicine Could Address Vaccine Hesitancy

Narrative medicine (NM) may be able to help us with a problem we share with the human medical community: a distrust and fear of vaccinations.

In an article in the journal *Human Vaccines & Immunotherapeutics* titled *Story and science: How providers and parents can utilize storytelling to combat anti-vaccine information*, the authors compare the tools used by the medical community to convince parents to vaccinate their children, namely "statistics, research, and other evidence-based information" with the method utilized by the antivaccine movement, which consists primarily of narratives. The article describes anti-vaccine social media pages, websites, and blogs which relate emotional stories of children who allegedly became sick after receiving a vaccination. Moderators often police comments and remove or berate those who are skeptical or disagree. The article authors conclude,

> With little or no science or evidence-based information to back up claims of vaccine danger, anti-vaccine activists have relied on the profound power of storytelling to infect an entire generation of parents with fear and doubt. And so some may argue that the success of the anti-vaccine movement is due to the fact that they have told a better story.
>
> (Shelby and Ernst 2013)

Yet all is not lost; the article recommends utilizing a combination of story and science to combat antivaccination bias. Providers can share positive vaccine experiences as well as stories of vaccine-preventable diseases (Shelby and Ernst 2013). In Chapter Five, we examined self-disclosure among pediatricians who discuss their own vaccination decisions as well as stories of clinical experiences with vaccine-hesitant parents; veterinary medicine may be able to implement similar NM strategies for dealing with vaccine-hesitant pet owners. The vaccine narrative may also be positively affected by the creation of the "vaccine selfie" to celebrate positive COVID-19 vaccination status.

On Being a New Veterinarian

Veterinary students and recent graduates may be concerned about being taken seriously by clients due to their inexperience and youthful appearance. It is important to remember not to take any skepticism personally and to consider the client's narrative. Pet owners are concerned about their animals and may be nervous about seeing someone new. Simply assure them that you will do your best to help their pet and move on with your exam. There's no need for a lengthy explanation about your experience.

It's also perfectly okay to acknowledge that you don't know something or that you'd like to look something up or check with a colleague before proceeding. Even if you feel as though you're doing it too often, the client has no idea how many times you've done so recently.

Case Story: *Have You Done This Before?*

As a new graduate, I sometimes had to work hard to earn a client's trust. When I noticed a skeptical look on a person's face, I tried hard to convert that look to, "she seems to know what she's talking about" by the end of the visit.

One clinic I worked at was owned by a 50-something male veterinarian, and clients were unused to seeing a 20-something female doctor. One day I saw a dog with multiple issues brought in by a female owner with a cynical expression. I addressed each issue, in turn, to the best of my ability, going over treatment scenarios in detail with the owner. By the end of the appointment, I was certain I had aced my "interview" and gained her trust. Last on the agenda was the expression of her dog's anal glands. As I inserted my gloved finger into the dog's rectum, the client asked, "Have you done this before?"

I learned there are some people you just can't please or convince, no matter what you say or do.

Practicing and Learning Through a Pandemic

This book was written during various stages of lockdown. Interviews were conducted over phone or Zoom, and as I complete the book, I haven't been in the same room as a client for an entire year, except for euthanasia appointments.

Some of the aspects of pandemic practice may continue in the future, such as an increased utilization of telemedicine and the option of curbside medicine. Going forward, we have the option to integrate parts of our pandemic narrative into our future one.

The pandemic has been an excellent time to put certain NM skills to the test. Here are some of them.

- Check Perfectionism at the Door – During the pandemic, most veterinary clinics were swamped, and client communication was frequently difficult. It was good practice for triaging and prioritizing the most important issues and concerns and occasionally leaving minor ones for the routine wellness exam. Did I mention the mild dental tartar accumulation to that client whose dog presented with lameness? I may not have. Normally, I would have. But during the pandemic, I was even more pressed for time. Communication was challenging. I needed to focus on making sure the owner understood the most important points. Besides, we weren't booking routine dentals at that point anyways, due to staffing issues from quarantines and childcare needs, and the local dental specialty clinic was booking out for months. Ideally, I'd still discuss the issue and let the client know we could address the teeth another time. But if I didn't, well, that was also okay. Is it the way I'd choose to practice? No. Was it acceptable, given the circumstances? Yes.
- Problem-Solve Creatively – At my workplace, two exam rooms (out of 5) have windows directly facing the parking lot. At the beginning of the pandemic, chief of staff Dr. Eileen Mulcahy decided to utilize the windows for communication. Chairs were set up about ten feet from the windows, along with a rope barrier six feet from the windows. Through the windows, clients were able to converse with the clinician, observe their pet's appointment, and reassure their animal verbally. It was as close as we could get to "normal," and although we still spoke to clients on the phone and in the parking lot, many of our interactions were through the windows.
- Try to Adjust – Clients love it when their vet compliments their animal. Normally, this is part of the ebb and flow of exam room conversation, beginning with greeting the client and pet. But when the client couldn't be in the exam room or at the window, I realized something was missing, so I tried to say something positive about the pet as soon as we got on the phone. The same comments I'd make in the room without thinking – *Look at that tail*! *I love his ears*! *She's so sweet*! *What a cute collar*! – seemed awkward at first when said over the phone, but they helped build a rapport with clients when we couldn't be together in person.

Practice Resilience – as Dr. Sonja Olson pointed out on a video session with veterinary students, anyone studying or practicing during the pandemic will be able to look back and remind themselves, *If I made it through that difficult time, I can make it through this too.* Many of us have learned to rely on our own unique coping skills and recognize that not every day can be a good day. Some days are just okay, and some are downright difficult. But tomorrow will be another day, and we can remember to be kind to ourselves and allow ourselves the same grace we give others.

Wanted: More NM Voices

In human medicine, there are many practitioners and authors in the field of NM, and veterinary narrative medicine (VNM) has room for many voices and opinions as well. VNM can grow both from looking to human NM and considering issues unique to veterinary medicine. There is much potential for NM to contribute to practice, from assisting with communication to informing our understanding of the human–animal bond, preventing compassion fatigue and burnout, and implementing a tradition of reflection to increase our enjoyment of our careers.

In March of 2021, the Massachusetts Veterinary Medical Association (MVMA) announced plans to feature a creative work from a member, whether artwork, photography, or writing, in each issue (Massachusetts Veterinary Medical Association 2021). Perhaps other newsletter will begin similar sections to help foster creativity in practitioners and an understanding that our work requires more than a knowledge of science.

The following case story was initially published in the MVMA Newsletter in February 2021, by author and MVMA Wellness Committee Chairperson Dr. Monica Mansfield.

Case Story: *A Story, a Name, and a Comfort,* by Dr. Monica Mansfield

Last year, pre-COVID, I attended a power-packed national veterinary well-being summit in Chicago with veterinary leaders, medical doctors, psychologists, and social workers. One of the keynote speakers was a well-known psychiatrist, Dr. Christine Moutier, who speaks nationally, including many television appearances and works hard in the suicide prevention and well-being field. She talked about how, years ago, she was given the job of helping turn around a famous medical school/hospital complex (UCSD) that had an extremely high suicide rate, about 13 people per year. This doctor, not exactly sure how to rectify this, struggled but implemented immediate changes that dealt with self-care and more humane work schedules. She created a culture that accepted vulnerability and valued the importance of self-compassion and at-the-ready counseling availability. The rate of distress among the medical residents and medical staff improved dramatically. In the ensuing 13 years that she was there, there was one more suicide (still too many), but not the same annual epidemic as before. One of the things Dr. Moutier spoke to us all about that stuck with me was the value of self-compassion, especially because so many medical professionals, human or animal, are prone toward perfectionism. And in the walk of self-nurturing, she suggested a strategy of having a secret gentle word to speak inside your head to yourself as if you were a young child in need of loving guidance. A name that you would want to be called yourself. The idea of this name is that you are easy on yourself within your own mind, the same way you would compassionately kneel down with a 5 year-old who had skinned their knee. From the podium, she mentioned what she calls herself and the name for herself she uses. At the time, I thought that was pretty brave for her in front of this huge group of scientific listeners. However, I thought about that and wondered what would I call myself? Interesting, but would I ever really use that? I tucked that untapped tidbit to the back of my mind.

Two months later, I attended a national music conference in New Orleans (Folk Alliance International) that is a full throttle, all-encompassing experience of music, thousands of people, industry meetings, more music, photography, and concerts large and small, planned and impromptu, that last through the wee hours of the night. After one of these late night small room sessions, I found myself with five or six musicians who had just played a spontaneous jam to close down the night in the room they hosted. I was witness to their music and after it was over, I gushed over how much I loved what they just did. As we spoke, one of the musicians made it clear to me that their own brilliant music came from a deep point of hurt from parents who had created a lot of trauma within this person, perhaps as generational remnants from their own fraught upbringings. My late night brain remembered the tucked away gem that Dr. Moutier, the psychiatrist on the stage in Chicago, had said in terms of self-compassion and having a gentle name for oneself. I brought that up to the several of us now gathered round in discussion; we went around the room and all picked the name we would each use for ourselves... no overthinking, just picking what sweetly came to mind. I started and picked the name Honey. The musician who told me of their struggles chose Tater. There was also Tadpole and Lala among these musically gifted adults. As we went around the room picking our names, I realized that was exactly the thing to do. At 3:30 in the morning, seven humans from different parts of the country with diverse life pathways were sharing their private childlike names with six other almost-strangers.

In this tumultuous year since that music conference, I have become quite close with one of those musician friends, and we periodically talk about Honey and Tater when some gentler path walking is needed. The prompts from me to my friend about "what would you say to Tater right now?" have kept this template forefront for me. Thankfully, quite recently my unplugged laptop spontaneously ignited on my lap – a sudden, very rare, unprovoked emergency that happened for no good reason. In that instant, I closed the lid and threw my laptop on the floor, and while smoke filtered out the sides of my laptop, I grabbed some oven mitts from the next room and raced the smoldering computer out our front door into the falling snow. A scare, but not a house fire. There is a burn mark on our wood floor, but no animals or humans or property damage occurred other than the computer carnage. I will soon be sent a replacement computer, but until then, I still don't know how much of my several years' worth of music photo editing is saved or what may be lost (backups exist but some projects will have to be rebuilt). While the event was scary and loss of creative work may exist, I think I was calm about the whole thing in the moment and afterward. I was talking later to a close friend who asked me what was going through my head as the computer caught on fire on my lap and how did I know what to do. In answering her, I realized that during the emergency, I gently spoke to Honey. In each step of the process, my brain spoke, "How good that you were paying attention," "You did a good job thinking to go get those oven mitts," "What a clever idea to put the computer out in the snow," "Great job, Honey!" I realized I had broken down each step I took into comforting words I would say to a child, and that helped me reframe what might otherwise have been a much more frightening experience. I think having practiced the tone with my friend made that kind of self-language a grace when I really needed it. And that is what made the laptop almost-fire event not become a psychic trauma event to me, thankfully.

So here is my recommendation and my conclusion. Let's give ourselves a gentle name. You already know mine. You already know those of some outstanding musicians from Louisiana and Nashville. No one ever needs to know yours if you wish. Or feel free to share yours with another person you trust. I feel like this inside-our-head name may be one key to self-compassion and self-cheerleading that can help you, and that is a very healthy thing" (Mansfield 2021).

Suggestions for Reflection and Discussion

- What does NM mean to you? In which directions would you like to see the field grow?
- How has the pandemic affected your practice or education?
- What subjects would you require if you were on a veterinary school admission committee?
- Based on Dr. Mansfield's story, choose a "gentle name" for yourself.

References

2011. *Project Implicit at Harvard*. Accessed March 15, 2021. https://implicit.harvard.edu/implicit/takeatest.html.

2017. "Jon Kabat-Zinn: Defining Mindfulness." *Mindful.org*. January 11. Accessed January 23, 2021. https://www.mindful.org/jon-kabat-zinn-defining-mindfulness/.

2020. "MCVMA.org." July 19. Accessed March 15, 2021. https://static1.squarespace.com/static/5e82bf22fa1955028bc37a61/t/5f14e47e8f488a75b5400c0b/1595204736191/Official+Statement+and+Actionables+for+the+AVMA+7-19-20.pdf.

2020. *Network Veterinary Humanities*. August 18. Accessed February 16, 2021. https://veterinary-humanities.blogspot.com/p/1st-conference-october-2020.html.

2021. "AAVMC Study Examines Bias in Admissions Processes, Standards." *Vet Med Educator: News from the AAVMC*. March.

Anderson J.G., Abrahamson K. 2017. "Your health care may kill you: Medical errors." *Stud Health Technol Inform*;234:13–17. PMID: 28186008.

Arbe Montoya A.I., Hazel S., Matthew S.M., McArthur M.L. 2019. "Moral distress in veterinarians…" *Vet Rec*;185(20):631. doi: 10.1136/vr.105289. Epub 2019 Aug 19. PMID: 31427407.

Arroll B., Allen E.C. 2015. "To self-disclose or not self-disclose? A systematic review of clinical self-disclosure in primary care." *Br J Gen Pract*;65(638):e609–16. doi: 10.3399/bjgp15X686533. PMID: 26324498; PMCID: PMC4540401.

AVMA@workblog. 2016. "Clarification regarding the New Graduate Starting Salary Calculator." May.

Babenko O., Guo Q. 2019. "Measuring self-compassion in medical students: Factorial validation of the self-compassion scale-short form (SCS-SF)." *Acad Psychiatry*;43(6):590–594. doi: 10.1007/s40596-019-01095-x. Epub 2019 Aug 8. PMID: 31396881.

Baggini J. 2015. "Euthanasia for Animals: What Can It Teach Us About Assisted Suicide in Humans?" *The Independent*, July 21.

Bain B., Ouedraogo F., Rosemary Radich M.A. 2020. *2020 Economic State of the Veterinary Profession*. AVMA.

Beach M.C., et al. 2013. "A multicenter study of physician mindfulness and health care quality." *Ann. Fam. Med.*;11(5): 421–8. doi:10.1370/afm.1507.

Becker M. 2015. "Why you should embrace fear free veterinary visits." *Veterinary Practice News*, June 9.

Becker M. 2016. "I lied when a pet died." *Veterinary Practice News*, February 2.

Begeny C.T., Ryan M.K., Moss-Racusin C.A., Ravetz G. 2020. "In some professions, women have become well represented, yet gender bias persists-Perpetuated by those who think it is not happening." *Sci Adv*;6(26):eaba7814. doi: 10.1126/sciadv.aba7814. PMID: 32.

Benson J., Magraith K. 2005. "Compassion fatigue and burnout: The role of Balint groups…" *Aust Fam Phys.*;34(6):497–8. PMID: 15931410.

Berkey F.J., Wiedemer J.P., Vithalani N.D. 2018. "Delivering bad or life-altering news." *Am Fam Phys*;98:99–104.

Bragg R.F., Bennett J.S., Cummings A., Quimby J.M. 2015. "Evaluation of the effects of hospital visit stress on physiologic variables in dogs." *JAVMA*;246(2):212–215.

Brandstetter G. 2020. "Program for Pet Health Equity." https://pphe.utk.edu. November. Accessed March 3, 2021. https://pphe.utk.edu/wp-content/uploads/2020/11/Public-Health-Guide.small_.pdf.

Bravata D.M., Watts S.A., Keefer A.L., Madhusudhan D.K., Taylor K.T., Clark D.M., Nelson R.S., Cokley K.O., Hagg H.K. 2020. "Prevalence, predictors, and treatment of impostor syndrome: A systematic review." *J Gen Intern Med*;35(4):1252–1275. doi:10.1007/s11606-019–05364.

Brown B. 2010. *The Gifts of Imperfection*. Center City, MN: Hazeldon Publishing, p. 55.

Brown B. 2019. "file:///C:/Users/kayrf/Downloads/Integration-Ideas_Emotional-Vocabulary.pdf page 2." *www.brenebrown.com*. August. Accessed January 21, 2021. file:///C:/Users/kayrf/Downloads/Integration-Ideas_Emotional-Vocabulary.pdf.

Centers for Disease Control and Prevention (CDC). 2020. *Cultural Competence In Health And Human Services*. October 21. Accessed December 23, 2020. https://npin.cdc.gov/pages/cultural-competence.

Chan M. 2020. "Pet owners are diverse, but veterinarians are overwhelmingly white. black veterinarians want to change that." *Time Magazine*, October 21.

Charon R. 2001. "Narrative medicine, a model for empathy, reflection, profession, and trust." *JAMA*;286:1897–1902.

Charon R. 2006. *Narrative Medicine, Honoring the Stories of Illness*. New York: Oxford University Press.

Charon R. 2017. *The Principles and Practice of Narrative Medicine*. New York: Oxford University Press.

Charon R., Wyer P. 2008. "Narrative evidence based medicine." *The Lancet*. doi:10.1016/s0140–6736(08)60156-7.

Childress M.D. 2017. "From doctors' stories to doctors' stories, and back again." *AMA J Ethics*;19(3):272–280. doi:10.1001/journalofethics.2017.19.3.nlit1-1703. PMID: 28323608.

Christianson A.L. 2002. "A piece of my mind. More stories." *JAMA*;288(8):931. doi:10.1001/jama.288.8.931. PMID: 12190350.

Cima G. 2020, "Social work expands in veterinar hospitals." *JAVMA* 1310–1313.

Coe J.B., O'Connor R.E., MacMartin C., Verbrugghe A., Janke K.A. 2020. "Effects of three diet history questions on the amount of information gained from a sample of pet owners in Ontario, Canada." *J Am Vet Med Assoc*;256:469–478.

Cook D.A., Sorensen K.J., Wilkinson J.M. 2014. "Value and process of curbside consultations in clinical practice: A grounded theory study." *Mayo Clin Proc*;89(5):602–14. doi: 10.1016/j.mayocp.2014.01.015. PMID: 24797642.

Crane M.F., Phillips J.K., Karin E. 2015. "Trait perfectionism strengthens the negative effects of moral stressors occurring in veterinary practice." *Aust Vet J*;93(10):354–60.

Delicano R.A., Hammar U., Egenvall A., Westgarth C, Mubanga M, Byberg L, Fall T, Kennedy B. 2020. "The shared risk of diabetes between dog and cat owners and their pets: register based cohort study." *BMJ*;371:m4337. doi: 10.1136/bmj.m4337. PMID: 33303475.

Diorio C., Nowaczyk M. 2019. "Half as sad: A plea for narrative medicine in pediatric residency training." *Pediatrics*;143(1):e20183109. doi: 10.1542/peds.2018-3109. Epub 2018 Dec 6. PMID: 30523202.

Every-Palmer S., Howick J. 2014. "How evidence-based medicine is failing due to biased trials and selective publication." *J Eval Clin Pract*;20(6):908–14. doi: 10.1111/jep.12147. Epub 2014 May 12. PMID: 24819404.

Fine K. 2018a. "Guide to Writing a Pet Obituary."

Fine K. 2018b. "How to Cope With a Serious Diagnosis." *Bark Magazine*. October.

Gantzer H.E., Block B.L., Hobgood L.C., Tufte J. 2020. "Restoring the story and creating a valuable clinical note." *Ann Intern Med*;173(5):380–382. doi:10.7326/M20-0934.

Gass J. LICSW, interview by Karen Fine. 2020. *Veterinary Social Worker* (November 30).

Gawande A. 2014. *Being Mortal: Medicine and What Matters in the End*. New York: Picador.

Gordon J. 2005. "Medical humanities: To cure sometimes, to relieve often, to comfort always." *Med J Aust* Jan 3;182(1):5–8. PMID: 15651937.

Gowda D., Dubroff R., Willieme A., Swan-Sein A., Capello C. 2018. "Art as sanctuary: A four-year mixed-methods evaluation of a visual art course addressing uncertainty through reflection." *Acad Med*;93:S8–S13.

Grigg E.K., Hart L.A. 2019. "Enhancing success of veterinary visits for clients with disabilities and an assistance dog or companion animal." *Frontiers in Veterinary Science* https://www.frontiersin.org/articles/10.3389/fvets.2019.00044/full, page 4.

Haldane S., Hinchcliff K., Mansell P., Baik C. 2017. "Expectations of graduate communication skills in professional veterinary practice." *J Vet Med Educ*;44(2):268–279. doi:10.3138/jvme.1215-193R.

Hammond J.A., Hancock J., Martin M.S., Jamieson S., Mellor D.J. 2017. "Development of a new scale to measure ambiguity tolerance in veterinary students." *J Vet Med Educ*;44(1):38–49. doi:10.3138/jvme.0216-040R. PMID: 28206843.

He B., Prasad S., Higashi R.T., Goff H.W. 2019. "The art of observation: A qualitative analysis of medical students' experiences." *BMC Med Educ*;19(1):234. doi: 10.1186/s12909-019-1671-2. PMID: 31242945; PMCID: PMC6595600.

Hobgood C., Sawning S., Bowen J., Savage K. 2006. "Teaching culturally appropriate care: A review of educational models and methods." *Acad Emerg Med*;13:1288–1295. doi:10.1197/j.aem.2006.07.031.

Holden C.L. 2020. "Characteristics of veterinary students: Perfectionism, personality factors, and resilience." *J Vet Med Educ*;47:488–496.

Jenicek M. 2006. "Evidence-based medicine: Fifteen years later. Golem the good, the bad, and the ugly in need of a review?." *Med Sci Monit*;12(11):RA241–51. PMID: 17072278.

Kahler S.C. 2015. "Moral stress the top trigger in veterinarians' compassion fatigue: veterinary social worker suggests redefining veterinarians' ethical responsibility." *J Am Vet Med Assoc*;246(1):16–8.

Klimecki O., Singer T. 2011. "Empathic distress fatigue rather than compassion fatigue? Integrating findings from empathy research in psychology and social neuroscience." In *Pathological Altruism*, by A. Knafo, G. Madhavan, D.S. Wilson and B. Oakley, 368–380. Oxford, New York: Oxford University Press.

Kogan L.R., Schoenfeld-Tacher R., Hellyer P., Grigg E.K., Kramer E. 2020. "Veterinarians and impostor syndrome: An exploratory study." *Vet Rec*;187(7):271.

Kosko J., Klassen T.P., Bishop T., Hartling L. 2006. "Evidence-based medicine and the anecdote: Uneasy bedfellows or ideal couple?." *Paediatr Child Health*;11(10):665–8. doi:10.1093/pch/11.10.665. PMID: 19030250; PMCID: PMC2528597.

Kubler-Ross E. 1969. *On Death and Dying*. New York: Simon & Schuster/Touchstone.

Kurtz S., Silverman J. 2005. *Teaching and Learning Communication Skills in Medicine*. Oxford, UK: Radcliffe Publishing.

Laor-Maayany R., Goldzweig G., Hasson-Ohayon I., Bar-Sela G., Engler-Gross A., Braun M. 2020. "Compassion fatigue among oncologists: the role of grief, sense of failure, and exposure to suffering and death." *Support Care Cancer*;28(4):2025–2031. doi:10.1007/s00520-019-05009-3.

Launer J. 2002. *Narrative-based Primary Care*. Boca Raton, FL: CRC Press.

Launer J. 2018. *Narrative-Based Practice in Health and Social Care*. New York: Routledge.

Lauren Bookbinder, DVM. 2021. April 4.

Lepere K., Etsekson N., Opel D.J. 2019. "Provider self-disclosure during the childhood vaccine discussion." *Clin Pediatr (Phila)*;58(6):691–695. doi:10.1177/0009922818817828. Epub 2018 Dec 5. PMID: 30516063.

Lewis A. 2020. *Access to care: 'Veterinary medicine's social justice issue'*. December 21. Accessed March 3, 2021. https://news.vin.com/default.aspx?pid=210&catId=-1&id=9954570.

Linder J.N. 2019. "5 ways mindfulness practice positively changes your brain." *Psychology Today*, May 9: https://www.psychologytoday.com/us/blog/mindfulness-insights/201905/5-ways-mindfulness-practice-positively-changes-your-brain#:~:text=5%20Ways%20

Mindfulness%20Practice%20Positively%20Changes%20Your%20Brain,Neural%20 Circuitry.%204%20Anterior%20Cingulate%20.

Little P., White P., Kelly J., et al. 2015. "Verbal and non-verbal behaviour and patient perception of communication in primary care: an observational study." *Br J Gen Pract*;65:e357–e365.

Lloyd J.W., Greenhill L.M. November 2020. *AAVMC Admissions: Report of 2019 Student Survey Analysis*. Research Analysis, AAVMC.

Maclaggan C. 2014. "Lack of hispanics in veterinary programs." *The New York Times*, August 14.

Magalhães-Sant'Ana M. 2019. "The emperor's new clothes-an epistemological critique of traditional chinese veterinary acupuncture." *Animals (Basel)*;9(4):168. doi:10.3390/ ani9040168. PMID: 30991678; PMCID: PMC6523156.

Malpass A., Binnie K., Robson L. 2019. "Medical students' experience of mindfulness training in the UK: Well-being, coping reserve, and professional development." *Educ Res Int*. doi:10.1155/2019/4021729. Epub 2019 Feb 3. PMID: 311684.

Mangione S., Chakraborti C., Staltari G., Harrison R., Tunkel A.R., Liou K.T., Cerceo E., Voeller M., Bedwell W.L., Fletcher K., Kahn M.J. 2018. "Medical students' exposure to the humanities correlates with positive personal qualities and reduced burnout: A multi-institutional U.S. survey." *J Gen Intern Med*;33(5):628–634. doi:10.1007/s11606-017-4275-8. Epub 2018 Jan 2.

Mansfield M. 2021. "A story, a name, and a comfort." *The MassVet News*, February: 11–12.

Mansfield M., DVM. 2021. April 10.

Massachusetts Veterinary Medical Association. 2021. "Highlight your talents in the newsletter." *MVMA Weekly Member Alert*, March 24.

Matte A.R., Khosa D.K., Coe J.B., Meehan M., Niel L. 2020a. " Exploring pet owners' experiences and self-reported satisfaction and grief following companion animal euthanasia." *Vet Rec*. doi: 10.1136/vr.105734. Epub ahead of print. PMID: 3249.

Matte A.R., Khosa D.K., Coe J.B., Meehan M., Niel L. 2020b. "Exploring veterinarians' use of practices aimed at understanding and providing emotional support to clients during companion animal euthanasia in Ontario, Canada." *Vet Rec*;187(9):e74. doi:10.1136/ vr.105659. Epub 2020 Apr 6. PMID: 32253355.

Matte A.R., Khosa D.K., Coe J.B., Meehan M.P. 2019. "Impacts of the process and decision-making around companion animal euthanasia on veterinary wellbeing." *Vet Rec*;185(15):480. doi:10.1136/vr.105540. Epub 2019 Aug 13. PMID: 31409747.

Mattson K. 2020a. "AVMA to launch certificate program promoting inclusive workplaces." *JAVMA*, December 1: 1095.

Mattson K. 2020b. "Veterinary social work summit focuses on animals, poverty." *JAVMA*, December 1: 1090–1091.

McDermott M.P., et al. 2015. "Veterinarian-client communication skills: current state, relevance, and opportunities for improvement." *J Vet Med Educ*;42(4): 305–14. doi:10.3138/ jvme.0115-006R.

McKenzie H.C., interview by Dr. Karen Fine. 2021. *Professor of Large Animal Medicine at Virginia-Maryland College of Veterinary Medicine* (January 11).

Meghani S.H., Byun E., Gallagher R.M. 2012. "Time to take stock: A meta-analysis and systematic review of analgesic treatment disparities for pain in the United States." *Pain Med*;13(2):150–74. doi:10.1111/j.1526-4637.2011.01310.x. Epub 2012 Jan 13. PMID: 2.

Meier B., Nietlispach F. 2019. "Fallacies of evidence-based medicine in cardiovascular medicine." *Am J Cardiol*;123(4):690–694. doi:10.1016/j.amjcard.2018.11.004. Epub 2018 Nov 24. PMID: 30527778.

Merriam-Webster. n.d. "Bechdel Test."

Montana B., interview by Dr. Karen Fine. 2021. *Vets4Vets Program Leader* (February 18).

Morris P. 2012. "Managing pet owner's guilt and grief in veterinary euthansia." *J Contemp Ethnogr*;41:337–365.

Mueller P.A., Oppenheimer D.M. 2014. "The pen is mightier than the keyboard: Advantages of longhand over laptop note taking." *Psychol Sci*;25(6):1159–68. doi:10.1177/0956797614524581.

Murphy J.W., Choi J.M., Cadeiras M. 2016. "The role of clinical records in narrative medicine: A discourse of message." *The Permanente J*;20:103–108.

Murphy J.W., Franz B.A., Schlaerth C. 2018. "The role of reflection in narrative medicine." *J Med Educ Curric Dev*.doi:10.1177/2382120518785301.

Nunez S. 2018. *The Friend*. Riverhead.

Ofri D. 2015. *Deconstructing our perception of perfection*. Performed by Dr. Danielle Ofri. Kennedy Center, Washington, D.C. May 12.

Ofri D. 2017. "Medical humanities: The Rx for uncertainty?" *Acad Med*;92(12):1657–1658. doi: 10.1097/ACM.0000000000001983. PMID: 28991847.

Pickersgill M.J., Owen A. 1992. "Mood-states, recall and subjective comprehensibility of medical information in non-patient volunteers." *Pers Individ Differ*;13(12):1299–1305.

Pontin E.E., Hanna J., Senior A. 2020. "Piloting a mindfulness-based intervention to veterinary students: Learning and recommendations." *J Vet Med Educ*;47(3):327–332. doi:10.3138/jvme.0618-076r. Epub 2019 Jun 13. PMID: 31194632.

Program for Pet Health Equity. Accessed March 3, 2021. https://pphe.utk.edu/.

Pun J.K.H. 2020. "An integrated review of the role of communication in veterinary clinical practice." *BMC Vet Res*;16(1):394. doi:10.1186/s12917-020-02558-2.

Remen R.N. 2016. *www.rachelremen.com*. Accessed September 21, 2020. http://www.rachelremen.com/about/.

Richman E., MSW, LICSW, interview by Karen Fine. 2020. *Veterinary Social Worker* (November 24).

Rochman S., interview by Karen Fine. 2021. *Social Worker* (March 25).

Ronald Epstein M.D. 2017. *Attending: Medicine, Mindfulness, and Humanity*. New York: Simon & Schuster.

Rowley S. 2016. *Lily and the Octopus*. New York: Simon & Schuster.

Sabin J.A. 2020. *Association of American Medical Colleges*. January 6. Accessed March 15, 2021. https://www.aamc.org/news-insights/how-we-fail-black-patients-pain.

Sackett D.L., et al. 1996. "Evidence based medicine: what it is and what it isn't." *BMJ (Clinical research ed.)*;312(7023):71–2. doi:10.1136/bmj.312.7023.71.

Shapiro T.R. 2015. "For veterinary students, the hardest lesson of all is saying goodbye." *the Washington Post*, September 26.

Shelby A., Ernst K. 2013. "Story and science: How providers and parents can utilize storytelling to combat anti-vaccine misinformation…" *Hum Vaccin Immunother*;9(8):1795–801. doi:10.4161/hv.24828. Epub 2013 Jun 28. PMID: 23811786; PMCID: PMC3906284.

Shmalberg J., Memon M.A. 2015. "A retrospective analysis of 5,195 patient treatment sessions in an integrative veterinary medicine service: Patient characteristics, presenting complaints, and therapeutic interventions." *Vet Med Int*;2015:983621. doi:10.1155/2015/983621.

Song S.J., Lauber C., Costello E.K., Lozupone C.A., Humphrey G., Berg-Lyons D., Caporaso J.G., Knights D., Clemente J.C., Nakielny S., Gordon J.I., Fierer N., Knight R. 2013. "Cohabiting family members share microbiota with one another and with their dogs." *Elife*;2:e0.

Suzuki S. 1970. *Zen Mind, Beginner's Mind*. Boulder: Shambhala.

Swede T.W., Marci J. 2016. "Transforming preprofessional health education through relationship-centered care and narrative medicine." *Teach Learn Med*;31:222–233.

Tayce J.D., Burnham S., Mays G., Robles J.C., Brightsmith D.J., Fajt V.R., Posey D. 2016. "Developing cultural competence through the introduction of medical spanish into the veterinary curriculum." *J Vet Med Educ*;43(4):390–397. doi:10.3138/jvme.0915-148R. Ep.

The Center For Culturally Proficient Educational Practice. n.d. *The Continuum*. Accessed December 23, 2020. https://ccpep.org/home/what-is-cultural-proficiency/the-continuum/.

Thompson D. 2013. "The 33 Whitest Jobs in America." *The Atlantic*, November 6.

Torppa M.A., Makkonen E., Mårtenson C., Pitkälä K.H. 2008. " A qualitative analysis of student Balint groups in medical education: contexts and triggers of case presentations and discussion themes." *Patient Educ Couns*;72(1):5–11. doi:10.1016/j.pec.2008.01.01.

Veterinary Social Work, The University of Tennessee Knoxville. Accessed January 28, 2021. https://vetsocialwork.utk.edu/.

Webb J.T., Gore J.L., Amend E.R., DeVries A.R. 2007. *A Parent's Guide to Gifted Children*. Tucson: Great Potential Press.

Whitaker D. 2021. "Proactive personal pronoun use: Creating a culture of inclusion in your practice." *Trends Magazine*, January: https://www.aaha.org/publications/trends-magazine/trends-articles/2021/mar-2021/proactive-personal-pronoun-use/.

Winkel A.F. 2016. "Narrative medicine: A writing workshop curriculum for residents." *MedEdPORTAL*;12:10493. doi:10.15766/mep_2374-8265.10493. PMID: 30984835; PMCID: PMC6440423.

Witte T.K., Kramper S., Carmichael K.P., Chaddock M., Gorczyca K. 2020. "A survey of negative mental health outcomes, workplace and school climate, and identity disclosure for lesbian, gay, bisexual, transgender, queer, questioning, and asexual veterinary professional." *JAVMA*;257:417–431.

Woolf S.H., George J.N. 2000. "Evidence-based medicine. Interpreting studies and setting policy." *Hematol Oncol Clin North Am*;14(4):761–84. doi:10.1016/s0889-8588(05)70310-5. PMID: 10949772.

Yazdankhahfard M., Haghani F., Omid A. 2019. "The Balint group and its application in medical education: A systematic review." *J Educ Health Promot*;8:124. doi:10.4103/jehp.jehp_423_18. PMID: 31334276; PMCID: PMC6615135.

Further Reading

The Spirit Catches You and You Fall Down: A Hmong Child, Her American Doctors, and the Collision of Two Cultures by Anne Fadiman

On Death and Dying by Elisabeth Kubler-Ross

Being Mortal by Atul Gawande

The Gifts of Imperfection by Brené Brown

Attending: Medicine, Mindfulness, and Humanity by Ronald Epstein

Narrative-Based Practice in Health and Social Care by John Launer

Narrative Medicine: Honoring the Stories of Illness by Rita Charon

The Immortal Life of Henrietta Lacks by Rebecca Skloot

The Radium Girls: The Dark Story of America's Shining Women by Kate Moore

Lily and the Octopus by Steven Rowley

Wicked by Gregory Maguire

Wonder by R. J. Palacio

Appendix A
Personal Loss Timelines, by Julie Gass, L.I.C.S.W.

Different types of losses occur during our lifespan and we don't always process them fully or even at all. These experiences are a part of our story and can impact how we deal with current loss. The act of creating a timeline provides a space for people to evaluate their losses, how they dealt with them at the time, and whether there is unfinished grief that needs to be addressed. My feelings as a grief counselor are that our society doesn't make much time for grief, and I would go as far as saying we want to shoo it away as soon as we are able. In this regard, it would make sense that people may not draw connections on how they are currently feeling to the past. Having a visual representation of your losses can help you see patterns in your past feelings and how you handled them, and maybe even how that time period in your life was impacted. Creating a timeline can increase self-awareness and gives you a tool to evaluate how you are currently dealing with grief. It works both ways... you can identify the strengths in your coping, and you can understand your vulnerabilities better as well.

The timeline I made is simple, but people can do it in a way that is unique to them. They can get more elaborate and, for instance, use symbols to represent relationships. I've seen some people use the thickness of the lines to indicate the intensity of the grief. Creating a timeline is something you can do by yourself or with a counselor as part of the grief intervention. The timelines remind me of ecomaps and genograms, which are also visual aids in understanding how your family relationships and environment shaped you.

Personal Loss Timeline - Sample

Personal Loss Timeline

[1976-1986]	[1987-1996]	[1997-2006]	[2007-2016]	[2017-]
1986 – Pet cat Oreo died	1994 -Left home for college in Virginia	2004 – Grandmother dies from CHF	2012 – Father diagnosed with prostate cancer	2020 – Covid 19 Pandemic
	1992 – Best friend got Lymphoma	2001 – Five year relationship ends	2007 – Parents sold childhood home	2019 – Childhood best friend dies
1982- Family moved to suburbs	1990 – Grandfather died from stroke	1999 – Graduated college	2005 – Married long-term boyfriend	2017 – Moved to Boston

Born 01/51976   2021-

| Oreo – Temporary sadness | Grandfather– Sadness, confusion Lymphoma – Anger, sadness, anxiety | Grandmother – Sadness, depression, guilt Break-up – Depression an | Sale of home – Regret, nostalgia, sadness Father – Fear, anxiety, anger, protective | Move – Anxiety, regret, excitement Death of friend – guilt sadness depression Pandemic – anger fear, depression |

Appendix B
Legacy Projects and Dignity Therapy, by Julie Gass, L.I.C.S.W.

Legacy projects are an intervention some mental health clinicians provide to families and human patients who are managing serious illness. They utilize various mediums, such as photos, music, talking, and art, to help patients and their families take stock of their lives and make meaning of them. Legacy projects help foster a sense of satisfaction in the accomplishments in one's life and can have powerful positive effects on the psychosocial symptoms that occur during end of life, such as loss of identity, anxiety, and depression. Dignity therapy is one example of a legacy project, where through a guided interview process, the patient discusses what is most important in their lives and what they are proud to leave behind. The conversation helps family and the medical care team see the patient as a culmination of their life and more than the illness they are experiencing. This helps clarify their individual needs in their medical care.

It would be beneficial to adapt some of these strategies for caregivers who are experiencing a serious illness with their animal companions. The satisfaction that comes along with reviewing shared life experiences can be helpful in goal-setting and end-of-life decision-making by aiding the client in honoring the happy life their pet led. It will also help them feel fulfilled in their role as a caregiver. The idea is that these feelings will ease the existential distress that comes with end-of-life decisions and insert more reassurance into an often ambiguous and heart-breaking process. Veterinarians may also benefit from legacy projects. Knowing more about the animal and the client they are working with will foster a deeper empathic relationship, which will facilitate communication and ease their own work-related stress by mitigating the anxiety that comes with end-of-life care.

Acknowledgments

When I've read long lists of thank-yous in acknowledgment sections, I've been amazed by the number of names listed. How does the author even *know* all those people? As it turns out, it really does take a village to write a book. I was fortunate to benefit from the generosity, expertise, and support of many people involved in the practice of both veterinary and human medicine.

Thank you to my wonderful editor Alice Oven for the opportunity to write this book, and to Damanpreet Kaur.

Thank you to Dr. Sonja Olson, Dr. Annie Wayne, Dr. Nick Frank, Karen Reagan, Dr. Lauren Bookbinder, Dr. Lynn Roy, Eric Richman MSW, LICSW, Julie Gass LICSW, Dr. Nancy Boren Alperson, Dr. Dane Whitaker, Dr. Alisha Matte, Dr. Éadaoin Redmond, Dr. Carol-Ann Farkas, Simon Rochman, Dr. Rita Charon, Dr. Katherine Nickerson, Dr. John Launer, Dr. Christina Tran, Dr. Harold C. McKenzie III, Dr. Lisa Schwartz, Dina Tedeschi, Dr. Ashley Emanuele, Mary E. Duane, Dr. Bree Montana, Jordan benShea, Dr. Marcia Day Childress, Dr. Robin Blumenthal, and Dr. Monica Mansfield.

Thank you to veterinary students and future colleagues Rachel Park, Elina Grunkina, Kayla Blyton, Kate O'Hara, Lauren Fay, Daniel Markstein, Catriona McIntyre, Michaela Roth, Kaneha Vali, Glenn Robbins, Sasha DiNitto, Rebecca Dreizen, and Asjah Fezio.

Thank you to the Seven Bridge Writers' Collaborative, Paula Castner, and the members of my writing critique group.

This book would not have been written without the shared reflections of my kindred questioning spirit, Dr. Eileen Mulcahy. Special thanks to my coworkers Cindy Moss and Michelle Cormier, and my entire work family at Central Animal Hospital in Leominster, Massachusetts.

Thank you to my husband Mike and son Nate (we might get our kitchen table back now!) for your humor and encouragement as well as Toffee, Sesame, and Lilac, for making me take frequent writing breaks. An extra thank you to Nate for creating the triangle diagrams! Thank you to David and Angela Fine for your endless support and advice and to Celia Fine for your encouragement and for raising a reader.

Index

Printed in the United States
by Baker & Taylor Publisher Services

Printed in the United States
by Baker & Taylor Publisher Services